Practical Physiotherapy for Veterinary Nurses

Practical Physiotherapy for Veterinary Nurses

Donna Carver BSc (Hons) Physiotherapy
Dip AVN (surg), RVN, MCSP

Chartered Physiotherapist, Specialist Veterinary Nurse
School of Veterinary Medicine
University of Glasgow, UK

WILEY Blackwell

Registered Office
John Wiley & Sons, Ltd, The Atrium, Southern Gate, Chichester, West Sussex, PO19 8SQ, UK

Editorial Offices
9600 Garsington Road, Oxford, OX4 2DQ, UK
The Atrium, Southern Gate, Chichester, West Sussex, PO19 8SQ, UK
1606 Golden Aspen Drive, Suites 103 and 104, Ames, Iowa 50010, USA

For details of our global editorial offices, for customer services and for information about how to apply for permission to reuse the copyright material in this book please see our website at www.wiley.com/wiley-blackwell

Library of Congress Cataloging-in-Publication Data

Carver, Donna, 1968– , author.
Practical physiotherapy for veterinary nurses / Donna Carver.
p. ; cm.
Includes bibliographical references and index.
ISBN 978-1-118-71136-1 (paper)
I. Title.
[DNLM: 1. Physical Therapy Modalities–nursing. 2. Physical Therapy Modalities–veterinary. 3. Hydrotherapy–veterinary. 4. Physical Examination–veterinary. 5. Veterinary Medicine–methods. SF 925]
SF925.C37 2016
636.089′5853–dc23

2015015321

A catalogue record for this book is available from the British Library.

Wiley also publishes its books in a variety of electronic formats. Some content that appears in print may not be available in electronic books.

Set in 9/12pt Meridien by SPi Global, Pondicherry, India

1 2016

Contents

Acknowledgements

I would like to dedicate this book to the patients and clients I have worked with throughout my career.

I would also like to thank the staff at the University of Glasgow Veterinary School for their support and for helping me make this book possible, with special thanks to Clare Skea (RVN) for her photography skills and patience.

About the companion website

Practical Physiotherapy for Veterinary Nurses is accompanied by a companion website:

www.wiley.com/go/carver/physiotherapy-veterinary-nurses

The website includes:

- Videos showing examples of exercises and treatments
- Self-assessment questions and answers taken from the book are offered in interactive form on the companion website to make testing yourself easier

CHAPTER 1

Musculoskeletal physiotherapy

Introduction

Gait analysis or assessment is a skill that requires close observation of the patient at walk and trot, to determine the cause and location of the lameness. A start point is to become familiar with a *normal* gait pattern, taking into account breed variations (i.e. dachshund vs bull mastiff). Once you are familiar with normal gait pattern, any deviation from this can be recognised.

Animals should be on a loose lead at walk and trot to observe for anatomical symmetry (normal gait pattern). Animals should be observed in a straight line towards, and then a straight line away from the observer. Pay particular attention to how the animal turns to both the left and right side – this may show reluctance to transfer weight onto the affected limb, or that the animal has issues with balance. The observer should then view the animal moving from both left and right sides. Subtle lameness may not readily be observed at walking pace; however, at trot the animal will only have one thoracic limb and one pelvic limb in contact with the ground, and these limbs will be placed under greater pressure meaning a lameness may be easier to detect.

Practical Physiotherapy for Veterinary Nurses, First Edition. Donna Carver.

Videoing the gait pattern, then slowing it down on playback, may be a useful way to detect lameness.

Gait analysis

Observe muscle symmetry, weight-bearing (paw and toe position) and conformation at rest.

Observe gait in a quiet area at walk and trot; thoracic limb lameness is often associated with head bobbing. When the animal takes its bodyweight through the painful thoracic limb the head will bob upwards in an attempt to unload the ground reaction force passing through the limb.

Pelvic limb lameness can be observed by a *hiking up* in the gluteal region in an attempt to offload or shift weight from the painful limb; this may be towards the contralateral pelvic limb, or forwards usually towards the contralateral thoracic limb. Lameness in pelvic limbs may also present with a *bunnyhopping* gait pattern. This may be related to a reduction in pelvic limb power, often observed with stair climbing or running. The bunnyhopping gait pattern may also be related to a reduced range of motion within the coxofemoral joint, which would be confirmed on physical examination.

Lameness is a general term used to describe an abnormal gait pattern; it may be:

Congenital – chondrodystrophic abnormalities, i.e. valgus (lateral deviation of the distal limb), often seen in dachshunds.

Or

Pathological – related to a disease process such as osteoarthritis, which can affect any breed but is often seen in larger breeds.

Scoring systems are often used to grade the degree of lameness, and in veterinary practice a typical 1–10 scale is used where 1/10 would indicate barely lame, whereas 10/10 would indicate non-weight-bearing lameness. The scale is very subjective, as only descriptive terms

Table 1.1 Lameness scoring scale.

Score	Description
0	Normal
1	Reduced weight-bearing through affected limb in stance
2	Mild lameness at trot
3	Moderate lameness at walk and trot
4	Intermittently carries limb, lame in trot
5	Non-weight-bearing lameness

From Summer-Smith (1993). Reproduced with permission from Elsevier.

are allocated to the very mildest and most severe lameness. If one observer rated lameness as 4/10, then a second observer may rate the same lameness as 6/10; does this indicate the lameness is progressing? This is why it is important to obtain a full and accurate history from the owner, who will probably observe the animal's gait every day and be able to state if the lameness is improving, staying the same, or deteriorating. A simpler alternative scoring 0–5 system is available (Table 1.1).

Elbow dysplasia gait analysis findings include abduction of the affected limb in an attempt by the patient to reduce the amount of bodyweight passing through the elbow joint. This will be most evident when the animal is ambulating on hard ground as the concussive forces passing through the elbow joint will be greater.

Flicking of the carpal joints is also evident with elbow dysplasia; this is a compensatory mechanism for the reduced range of motion, especially elbow flexion, that is characteristic of advanced elbow dysplasia. The condition is often bilateral, so it is important to observe how the animal turns (weight transfer) and observe (or ask the owner about) functional activities such as how or if the animal is able to descend stairs or jump from the car; this will increase load on the elbow joint and will be uncomfortable for the animal so he may avoid these functional activities.

Hip dysplasia gait analysis findings may include a short stride length; this is usually shown as reduced hip extension and can be readily observed as the animal climbs stairs as a weak or short hip extension/push-off. The reduction in hip extension is a characteristic of hip dysplasia, with associated osteoarthritis and joint remodelling.

Adduction of the affected limb is also evident. This can be due to weakness in the hip flexor muscle groups, and may also be associated with secondary osteoarthritic changes and compensatory coxofemoral joint remodelling. As discussed earlier *hiking up* of the gluteals to shift bodyweight from the affected limb, and *bunnyhopping* with bilateral hip dysplasia are also gait characteristics observed with this disease.

Cruciate rupture patients usually present with an abnormal gait pattern. Lameness can vary from mild 1/5 (usually chronic) to 5/5 (usually acute). The degree of lameness often correlates with the level of pain the animal is experiencing. A short stride length, especially reduced extension, is evident; also the animal will tend to limit stifle flexion. The animal will usually guard or resent stifle end-of-range flexion. *Clicking* of the joint may be evident and may indicate associated meniscal damage; this may be evident when the animal flexes the stifle joint, and loads the joint with bodyweight, such as in stair climbing. In acute presentation a joint effusion may be present. In chronic presentations thickening of the joint on the medial surface often with a tibial buttress is common. Stifle range of motion (ROM) is reduced as a result of scar tissue formation and secondary osteoarthritic changes.

The animal may abduct the limb to alter the direction of ground reaction forces passing through the joint, and if there is fatigue or weakness in the hip flexor muscle groups.

The animal will be reluctant to fully weight-bear through the affected limb; at rest, toe touch weight-bearing is often evident; the animal may also adopt various strategies to reduce weight-bearing in stance and will often position the affected limb in a cranio-medial plane.

The long-term muscle changes associated with pelvic limb lameness are short, tight hip flexor muscles, with, weak hamstring muscles. The goal for the physiotherapist is to stretch the short, tight muscles, whilst strengthening the weak, muscles.

History taking

This should include:

1 Age – *Young dogs*: When taking a history consider hip dysplasia, elbow dysplasia, oesteochondrosis dissecans (OCD).
Adult dogs: Consider osteoarthritis, cruciate disease and neoplasia.

2 Breed – *Toy breed*: Often show patella luxation, Legg–Calvé–Perthes disease.
Large breed: May present with cruciate disease, elbow dysplasia, neoplasia.

3 Onset of lameness:
- **a** May be sudden or subtle or traumatic.
- **b** Can be episodic or cyclic.
- **c** Is it consistently the same limb or a shifting lameness?

4 Duration of lameness:
- **a** Can be continuous or intermittent.
- **b** Is the patient's condition deteriorating, remaining static or improving?

5 Association:
- **a** Does exercise or rest effect the condition?
- **b** Does the patient appear worse in the morning or night?
- **c** Is there a seasonal pattern when symptoms are seen in summer or winter?
- **d** Does soft or hard ground affect the severity of symptoms?

6 Behavioural changes:
- **a** Is the patient showing aggression?
- **b** Does the patient have sleep disturbance?
- **c** Is the patient reluctant to play/jump?

7 Exercise – Ask about type, frequency and duration.

8 Response to treatment:
  a Is the patient on any medication, has this made any difference?
  b Has the patient had any previous physiotherapy treatment? If so what was the response or outcome?
  c Explore the owner's expectations of physiotherapy.

Physical examination

When assisting with a physical examination try to find a quiet area. Adopt a systematic anatomical approach each and every time. With the animal standing each limb will be lifted in turn to gauge weight-bearing through the limbs. Obviously the animal will be taking least weight through the affected limb, but lifting each limb in turn may give an indication of where the animal is shifting his bodyweight as a compensatory measure. Compensatory measures can often lead to secondary musculoskeletal issues so these should be noted during the physical exam and addressed later.

When assessing muscle mass compare with the unaffected contralateral limb for muscle mass symmetry. A standard tape measure can be used to measure the circumference of muscle bulk. Again, try to be systematic to ensure accuracy. For example, when measuring pelvic limb muscle bulk try to measure in standing, measure at the thickest point – this usually corresponds to the level of the muscle belly. Try to have a landmark – say in the pelvic limb the greater trochanter of the femur – where the two ends of the tape measure should meet and record the measurement. A difference of more than 1 cm would be considered significant. It is good practice to measure three times and take the average measure from the three readings and record this average reading in the notes.

Conscious proprioception may be delayed or absent in the presence of a joint effusion, which is often evident in acute cranial cruciate ligament injury.

Exercise plans

Exercise plans are designed to rehabilitate patients back to their highest level of function; they can be staged and should be progressive:

- *Early phase* (approximately 0–2 weeks): this time scale will depend on the patient's condition. The aims will be to control inflammation, maintain joint ROM and muscle length.
- *Mid-phase* (approximately 2–6 weeks): during this phase the patient should be progressing. The aims are to build on the progress from the early phase and also to improve strength, balance and proprioception.
- *Late phase* (approximately 6–12 weeks): this stage is when the patient will continue to gain strength, regain balance and improve stamina.

Early stage post-surgical rehabilitation will begin on day 1 postoperatively. Aim to minimise pain and inflammation, ensure non-weight-bearing (NWB) status on affected limb, maintain joint ROM and muscle length.

Mid-stage rehabilitation can commence 14 days postoperatively, following a satisfactory check-up from the veterinary surgeon and suture removal. The aims are to begin to increase joint ROM of the affected limb, and increase muscle length and mass on the affected limb. Begin gentle partial weight-bearing (PWB) exercises to increase function and strength, and prevent secondary compensatory postures and complications from developing.

Late-stage rehabilitation can commence at 6 weeks postoperatively following a satisfactory check-up from the veterinary surgeon, who may take survey radiographs at this stage to check healing. Rehabilitation goals will be to continue to strengthen the muscles of the affected limb. The patient may be full weight-bearing (FWB) on the affected limb at this stage.

Commence balance and proprioceptive exercise training using wobble cushions, wobble boards and cavaletti pole work. Address compensatory postures, which may be associated with trigger points.

Address secondary complications such as muscle imbalances (tight in flexor muscle groups, weak in extensor muscle groups, which is a common finding in animals with long-term lameness). Finally, the aim of the rehabilitation programme is to return the patient back to the highest level of function, so late-stage rehabilitation will address cardiovascular fitness or stamina, which will have been effected by the graded return to function rehabilitation programme.

Also consider the owner's ability and commitment to carry out the rehabilitation programme, plus environmental factors. The owner may work full time and have other family commitments. The rehabilitation home exercise programme should fit in with the animal's needs and the owner's time restrictions. Do not advise a rehabilitation home exercise programme that takes any more than 30 minutes twice daily to ensure owner compliance. Environmental factors to consider would include: are there other animals in the house, and are there stairs in the house that the patient needs to use?

Physiotherapy treatment techniques and modalities

Cold therapy

Cold therapy aims to control and minimise inflammation postoperatively or following acute injury. The body responds to injury by triggering an inflammatory reaction in the cells. The normal inflammatory phase in healthy tissues is approximately 72 hours. This is the period of time when cold therapy is recommended to minimise the inflammatory response.

Signs of inflammation

- *Pain* – from swollen or damaged nerve endings.
- *Redness* – from damage of local tissues.
- *Heat* – from dilation of local blood vessels.
- *Swelling* – from the associated capillaries becoming more permeable resulting in oedema of the local area.

Cold can be applied to the affected area in several ways. Broken ice chippings wrapped in a plastic zip-lock bag covered by a damp cloth, applied to the affected area for 10–20 minutes can be effective. This treatment can be repeated every 4–6 hours as required.

Usually begin the treatment early to minimise the inflammatory response. If an animal is recovering from surgery and is hypothermic, treatment may be postponed until the patient's body temperate returns to normal.

Cold therapy works by causing vasoconstriction of the local damaged blood vessels, thereby reducing swelling, damage to local tissues, and oedema.

Contraindications

- Cold hypersensitivity.
- Altered skin sensation.

Cautions

- Cardiac conditions.
- High blood pressure.
- Open healing wounds.
- Areas over superficial nerves.

Heat therapy

Various methods can be used to apply heat to the superficial tissues, such as wheat bags and heat discs that can be warmed in the microwave. Alternatively a damp towel can be microwaved, placed in a zip-lock bag and applied to the affected area for 10–20 minutes. This can be repeated every 4–6 hours.

Heat therapy can commence once the inflammatory phase has passed (usually 72 hours post-injury).

The principle of heat therapy is to vasodilate local blood vessels thus increasing blood flow to the local area to promote healing. Increased cellular activity results in an increase of oxygen and nutrients delivered to the cells.

Heat therapy can be used to reduce pain, stiffness and muscle spasm. Heat improves the elasticity of tissues and can be use prior to stretching.

Contraindications

- Sensory changes.
- Burns/scalds.
- Thrombus/embolism.
- Hyper- or hypo-sensitivity to heat.
- Infections.
- Malignant tumours.

Positioning and supports

Positioning aids and supports are used to maintain muscle length and support the weight of the affected limb. The animal may not have full function or control of the affected limb postoperatively. This may be exacerbated by factors such as pain or discomfort, bulky dressings or external fixators.

The animal will usually choose not to lie on the same side as the affected limb. However, the animal may find it difficult to find a comfortable position in which to rest. In most circumstances the animal will be more comfortable if the affected limb is supported in a neutral position, or slightly elevated in the early stages of recovery, and this will also prevent any muscle imbalances from developing. Folded beds, towels and pillows can be used to maintain the required position. Gentle handling and support of the affected limb and reassuring the animal are essential to aid compliance.

If a patient is placed with the injured limb uppermost and appears uncomfortable, or if the animal continually changes his position to lie on the injured limb, leave the animal in this position as he obviously finds it more comfortable. However, it is preferable not to allow the animal always to lie on one side, so attempt to gently reposition the animal on his non-affected side even if he only tolerates this position for a short period.

Ensure that if the patient's trunk is positioned in sternal recumbency and the patient has a support at his lateral thorax so he is not weight-bearing excessively or unevenly through his elbow joints. Ensure the elbows are equally abducted to prevent uneven weight-bearing, which could result in pressure sores. If the affected limb is positioned uppermost an adductor wedge or internal rotator wedge should be placed between the limbs to prevent muscle imbalance – for instance, weak gluteals versus tight adductors. Aim to use the adductor wedge to place the affected limb in a neutral position as this will be most likely tolerated by the patient.

Many waterproof animal mattresses are available to assist in preventing pressure sores. However, this will create an unstable surface when the animal is standing, and walking in and out of the kennel. Position yourself on the opposite side of the affected limb when assisting the patient to stand and walk in and out of the kennel. When positioned on the unaffected side you are able to assist the animal to shift his weight onto his unaffected limb to ensure he does not lose his balance.

Manual aids

Slings

Slings are used to assist the animal when he is mobilising. A variety of slings are available for veterinary use, most commonly used with orthopaedic patients is The Soft Quick Lift™ (Four Flags Over Aspen, Inc.) abdominal sling. This type of sling is useful following pelvic limb surgery, is easy to use, and is usually well tolerated by the patient. If you are using a sling to assist the patient to mobilise, position yourself on the same side as the unaffected limb in line with the pelvic limb. In this position you can tilt the patient slightly onto his unaffected limb and assist with balance if necessary and prevent him from falling.

In the early stages following orthopaedic surgery it is not desirable for a patient to weight-bear on the affected limb. This is because the soft tissues and bones are still healing, stabilising and remodelling. *Early weight-bearing is not a sign of successful surgery*. The sling is used in much the same way that a human would use crutches following surgery to a pelvic limb. The crutches are used to *protect* the limb whist healing takes place until a bony callus forms; the implant used to stabilise the joint is not strong enough to allow the individual to bear full weight through the affected limb.

A Helping Hand pelvic support sling (Mikki, Dorking, Surrey, UK) is sometimes used to support orthopaedic patients postoperatively when they are mobilising. A Helping Hand can be more difficult to place on the patient, it may be easier to assist the patient to stand, then whilst supporting him, position his feet in the limb holes of the Helping Hand and then pull them up, secure with Velcro and fasten the clips.

A Helping Hand sling is preferred to The Soft Quick Lift™ sling for animals undergoing pelvic or hip surgery as it gives added support to the pelvis and does not *block* hip flexion movements. A Helping Hand sling would also be the support aid of choice for thoracic limb post-surgical support. Given that the dog bears 60% of his bodyweight through the thoracic limbs support of the thoracic limbs to allow healing to take place is even more crucial.

For animals with multiple trauma to several limbs a fully body sling and mobile hoist may be necessary to assist mobilisation. The body sling supports the animal's trunk, whereas the hoist supports the animal's bodyweight; the hoist is slowly moved forwards and the animal can move his limbs without taking very much of his body weight.

Electrotherapy

Electrotherapy can be a useful modality when used in conjunction with therapeutic rehabilitation exercises.

Pulsed electromagnetic energy (PEME; Biomag® therapy)

The unit consists of a control panel and an electronic waterproof pad that can be placed under the affected area to be treated. It is a non-invasive treatment and as such is usually well tolerated by the patient. It is especially useful for treatment in arthritic patients and uses pulsed magnetic therapy to reduce pain and inflammation. PEME can be used in both the acute and chronic phases of disease. Pulsed magnetic therapy has been used in the assistance of bone healing.

Class IV laser

This can be used to treat wounds, for chronic and acute musculoskeletal conditions, for soft tissue injures, for pain and to control oedema (Figure 1.1). Power settings and the duration of treatment are calculated according to species, skin colour, bodyweight, area to be treated and the stage of the condition (acute or chronic). *N.B. Eyes must be protected with dark-green lens glasses.*

Contraindications of laser therapy

- Do not use laser therapy in pregnant animals.
- Do not use laser therapy to treat animals' eyes.
- Do not use laser therapy in animals with neoplasia.
- Do not use laser therapy over the thyroid area.

Transcutaneous electrical nerve stimulation (TENS)

This consists of a small control box, with wires leading to electrode pads. It is used to reduce pain by transmitting small electrical pulses to the affected area via the electrode pads.

The transcutaneous electrical nerve stimulation (TENS) machine can be used at a frequency of 90–130 Hz to stimulate large nerve fibres that activate the inhibitory interneurons that block the signal in the projection neurons that connect to the brain, and thereby blocking pain perception. If small nerve fibres become active and stimulate

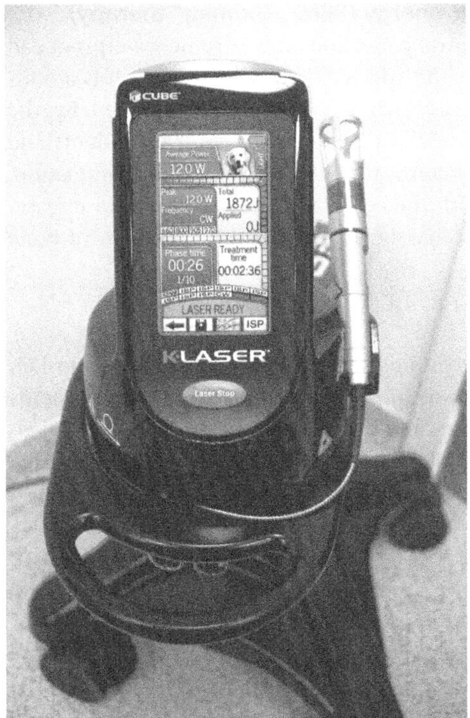

Figure 1.1 The K-Laser™ programmed and ready to use on a patient.

the projection neurons, this blocks the inhibitory interneurons and pain will be perceived in the brain.

When the TENS machine is set at a frequency of 2–5 Hz this stimulates the body to produce its own pain-easing chemicals, endorphins, thereby blocking the pain signals.

Many research studies have investigated the positive effects of TENS in humans with orthopaedic and neurological conditions. One study (Millis & Levine, 2014) investigated the effect of TENS on osteoarthritic pain in the stifle of dogs. Five dogs with chronic mild osteoarthritis, induced by cranial cruciate ligament resection and stifle stabilisation, were treated with TENS stimulation (70 Hz) applied to the affected stifle. Pre-treatment ground reaction forces were determined using a force plate before electrical stimulation to assess the functional use of the limb.

Significant improvements in ground reaction forces were found 30 minutes after treatment. These differences persisted for 210 minutes after TENS application and were statistically significant 30, 60, 120 and 180 minutes after treatment.

Each dog was re-evaluated following a 4-day rest period and still exhibited a mild increase in weight-bearing on the affected limb, but these differences were not significant. The author concluded this preliminary study showed positive benefits of TENS application in dogs with osteoarthritic stifle joints.

Manual techniques

Passive range of motion exercises

Passive range of motion (PROM) exercises are movements usually of the limbs performed by an individual such as a physiotherapist. The joints of the limbs are moved passively, and the patient does not gain any *strengthening* benefits from passive movements of the limbs.

PROM exercises are performed to maintain or improve joint ROM, and to prevent joint inflammation and stiffness. PROM exercises are especially important in recumbent animals that may already have established osteoarthritis and associated pain, stiffness and reduced ROM in the affected joints.

If the patient has undergone joint surgery full ROM of the joint is neither desirable nor essential in the early stages. However, full ROM should be maintained in all the other joints of the affected limb.

PROM exercises can commence from day 1 postoperatively. Gentle PROM exercises within the pain-free range will assist with lymphatic drainage of the limb and limit oedema when used in conjunction with positioning. If the distal limb is oedematous, compression followed by release exercises can be performed: two sets of 50 repetitions appear to be effective.

As the inflammatory phase passes PROM exercise of the affected joint may be gradually increased within the pain-free range, and with consent from the veterinary surgeon.

The animal is usually recumbent for the PROM exercises with the affected limb(s) uppermost. (However, the exercises can be performed in standing with the patient supported.) If the animal has undergone joint surgery this joint should be isolated and gently moved through its pain-free range in all anatomical planes. This joint would then be supported and the other joints in the affected limb would be moved through full ROM in all anatomical planes. PROM exercise three sets of 10 repetitions for each joint twice a day is considered to be effective.

If the patient has not undergone joint surgery and the PROM exercises are being performed to reduce pain, inflammation and stiffness in the joint, all the joints in the limb can passively be moved together. Be aware that if the patient has established osteoarthritis, ROM in the joint may be reduced and at the end of range you will feel a *bony block*; *do not* force the joint beyond this point as it will cause the patient further discomfort.

When performing PROM exercises the movements of the operator will push the joints together and then push them apart. PROM exercises should *never* involve pulling a limb or joints. Do not grip the limb tightly. If all joints are to be moved together into flexion then extension the patient should be supported at the medial elbow for the thoracic limb, and at the medial stifle for the pelvic limb to prevent any rotation of the joints, which may be uncomfortable. The movements should be in line with normal anatomical planes of movement (Table 1.2).

Stretches

Stretches are performed to maintain or increase muscle length. These are usually performed passively by an operator for recumbent patients, or in patients that have undergone surgery.

Table 1.2 Normal canine joint range of motion.

Joint	Degrees of movement
Carpus	Flexion 20–35° Extension 190–200° Valgus 10–20° Varus 5–15°
Elbow	Flexion 20–40° Extension 160–170°
Shoulder	Flexion 20–40° Extension 160–170° Abduction 40–50° Adduction 40–50°
Tarsus	Flexion 40° Extension 170°
Stifle	Flexion 45° Extension 160–170°
Hip	Flexion 55° Extension 160–165°

If a muscle crosses two joints, such as the quadriceps, any shortening of this muscle group will affect the ROM of the hip and stifle joint. As the quadriceps muscle group shortens, the stifle and hip will be brought into flexion. If the quadriceps becomes shortened or contracted for a prolonged period of time the patient will be unable to extend the stifle and hip, and so weight-bearing through the limb will become problematic.

Changes in muscle length can occur quickly in: (i) recumbent animals; (ii) patients that have recently undergone surgery when they may not be moving limbs through their full ROM; or (iii) an animal that is non-weight-bearing for a period of time, when the flexor muscles will become short and tight, and the opposing extensor muscle groups will become weak.

In recumbent animals stretches should begin on day 1. Flexor, extensor and internal rotator muscle groups should be stretched at least twice daily. Each stretch is held for 15 seconds, the animal is given a few seconds to rest, then the stretch is repeated three times in total. Following stretches, if the patient is resting in lateral recumbency, a wedge should be placed between the thoracic and pelvic limbs to prevent adductor/abductor muscle imbalance. Recumbent animals tend to become tight in the adductor muscle groups, and weak in the abductor muscle groups. Correct positioning following stretches can help to prevent muscle imbalance from occurring.

Stretches can be performed with the patient lying laterally or in standing. If the stretches are performed in standing, the animal will need to be supported at the trunk. The operator will use one hand to support at the origin of the muscle being stretched; with other hand a pushing force will be applied at the insertion of the muscle. The muscle should be stretched until resistance is felt in the muscle, then at this point the stretch should be *held* for 15 seconds and repeated three times. Stretching should not be uncomfortable for the patient. As described earlier pre-warming a muscle will improve the elasticity of the tissues, thus improving the range of the stretch. This may be useful if the animal is cold, has muscle spasm or has developed muscle contractures.

Mobilisations

Mobilisations are graded movements or manipulations of joints that are passive and usually performed by a physiotherapist.

The grade of movement delivered depends on the desired effect of the mobilisation or manipulation. For example, a grade II mobilisation would be a repetitive movement of a joint within its pain-free range with the aim of relieving pain within the joint. However, a grade III mobilisation would also be a repetitive movement of a joint but greater force would be applied with the aim of increasing ROM within that joint.

Mobilisations are treatments used to maintain ROM in painful joints; once the pain within the joint is manageable the grade of mobilisation can be increased to increase ROM within stiff joints.

The operator will be positioned close to the patient. If, for example, the joint mobilisation is to be applied to the spinal processes of the lumbar spine to increase extension the patient will preferably be lying in sternal recumbency. The operator will position her or his hands so that one thumb overlaps the other and using a pulsing motion pressure will be applied directly to the spinal process. *The physiotherapist is aligned over the patient and the pressure transmits from the shoulders down the arms to the thumbs; if the pressure was generated from the thumbs alone the physiotherapist would fatigue quickly.*

In conjunction with passive exercises to improve ROM and passive stretches to increase muscle length, progressive exercise programmes focused around the assessment findings can be useful adjuncts to achieve short- and long-term goals.

Progressive exercise programmes

1 Begin with gentle passive and progressive PROM exercises; aim to work within the pain-free range. Repeat the PROM flexion/extension exercises for three sets of 10 repetitions.

   Consider the use of electrotherapy such as a class IV K-Laser™, if available, to reduce pain and inflammation within the joint and control scar tissue, which may reduce ROM.

   If available hydrotherapy using an underwater treadmill (UWT) would be an ideal active exercise for the patient to increase ROM of the joint. Use the buoyancy effect of the water and fill to the level of the patient's mid-trunk. Start with slow speeds and short duration with plenty of rest breaks, then increase speed and time as the patient progresses.

2 Stretch short/tight muscles into early resistance, and hold each stretch for 15 seconds, then allow the patient to relax and repeat the stretch, for a total of three stretches. As the patient progresses with his exercise programme he will be functionally stretching

muscles as he ambulates and increases weight-bearing through the limb. Controlled stair climbing with support or ascending gentle slopes will all functionally stretch muscles.

3 Gently start to gradually increase weight-bearing on the affected limb by using weaving exercises to encourage weight transfer onto the affected limb. Start with the cones wide apart; to progress the exercise over the 6-week period reduce the distance between the cones, increase the speed of the exercise (tempting the patient with a treat may help), and gradually towards the end of the 6-week period reduce the support given by the sling.

   Hydrotherapy using a UWT can also be used to strengthen the extensor muscles as the patient places his limb in the stance phase and pushes through the limb and enters the swing phase. As the patient progresses a faster belt speed will encourage longer strides and greater activity in the extensor muscle groups.

4 Inflammation within the joint may affect conscious proprioception (CP). Stepping over cavaletti poles will challenge and improve CP as the patient will need to think about where he is placing his limb once he clears the pole. Start with the poles low and wide apart, progress by increasing the height and number of poles. Progress him further by altering the arrangement of poles (high, low, high, low).

   Exercising him on different surfaces will improve his CP, as on a slightly uneven surface he will receive increased afferent feedback from his foot to his brain signalling how he should place his foot. Start by exercising him on flat, firm, non-slip surfaces and progress him to grass, bark chippings and sand, which will be the most challenging surface.

   Practising functional activities in a controlled environment will boost the animal's confidence to carry out these activities in the home environment. If the animal has stairs to negotiate in the home or other places he visits this activity should be practiced under supervision.

   Stair climbing is a functional activity that requires strength to ascend the stairs, and balance to descend the stairs (Figure 1.2).

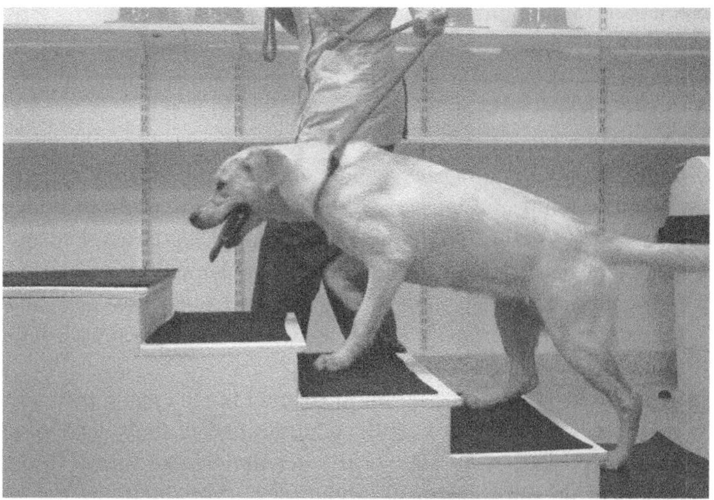

Figure 1.2 A patient ascending stairs. Note the reciprocal gait pattern: the right thoracic limb is flexed to step up, and the left pelvic limb is extended to push off onto the step. The right pelvic limb is flexed to place the limb on the stair, and the left thoracic limb is extended as weight is being taken through this limb.

Another common functional activity that the animal may need to perform is getting in and out of the car. A ramp is recommended for medium to large dogs. If the animal has not used the ramp before he may be reluctant to use it. Always make sure the ramp is firmly secured to the car. Start by practising getting into the car first so he can gain confidence. Practice this several times before attempting using the ramp to exit the car. Like with stair practice he will feel most vulnerable on the descent. It may be useful to have an assistant at the opposite side of the ramp to yourself to give extra reassurance and to assist the patient should he lose his balance.

Early gait re-education is vital to prevent any secondary complications or compensatory postures from developing. If the animal is holding the limb in extreme hip flexion most of the time he is at risk of developing muscle imbalance (tight in flexors vs weak in extensors). He is also at risk of developing severe muscle atrophy in the extensor muscle groups, and reduced joint ROM.

Another point to note is the extra pressure placed on the other limbs, mainly the other pelvic limb and the contralateral thoracic limb. The joints and muscles in these limbs will be placed under greater stress so function in these limbs should also be assessed and treated as necessary. Also the lumbar spine should be assessed in pelvic limb chronically lame animals for any signs of stiffness, and for pain in the associated muscles, which may develop muscle tension or *trigger points*.

Laser therapy can be useful in treating lumbar spine pain and inflammation associated with chronic pelvic limb lameness. Alternatively, or as an adjunct to laser therapy treatment, direct ischaemic pressure treatment can be used at the site of the trigger point. A *gradual* pressure equating to approximately 4 kg is applied until the trigger point or muscle spasm diminishes.

Lumbar spine pain and stiffness can be treated with mobilisations. Start gently with grade II for pain relief, then progress to grade III to improve mobility and reduce stiffness.

Active-assisted (using a sling) exercises in a controlled environment are an excellent way to reduce gait abnormalities. As the patient is challenged by the exercises (weaving cones/cavaletti poles) he will not be able to compensate by mobilising on three limbs and therefore will commence with gentle weight-bearing, which is desirable at this stage of the rehabilitation programme.

5 Hydrotherapy using a UWT is another excellent exercise to improve gait abnormalities as the buoyancy of the water means the patient will have less weight and concussive forces passing through his joints so he will be more likely to use the limb. The warmth of the water will also assist in relaxing any muscle tension. The speed, duration (time), and level of the water (buoyancy effect) can all be

controlled to suit the needs of the patient and the rehabilitation programme. Start with slow speeds and short duration; it is important that the patient gains confidence to begin with.

The aim of the late-stage rehabilitation programme is to *fine tune* any minor discrepancies regarding joint ROM or muscle imbalances. The late-stage programme aims to improve strength of the affected limb, improve muscle bulk, improve CP and balance, and finally to improve stamina.

1 *Balance*: simply start by testing the patient's ability to resist perpetrations or 'nudges', forcing the patient to take weight through the affected limb(s). This exercise can be progressed to incorporate limb lifting. Start by lifting the affected limb, then progress to lifting the non-affected pelvic limb (support the patient as necessary with an arm under his abdomen at the start). Progress the exercise by lifting the contralateral thoracic limb (diagonal lifting). Hold each limb lift for 5 seconds and repeat five times.

   A wobble cushion can be placed under the patient's limb. Perpetrations or nudges at the contralateral hip will force the patient's limb onto the wobble cushion, which is an unstable surface so he will need to use stabilising muscles in the limb to maintain his balance. If this exercise is well tolerated, it can be progressed by incorporating limb lifting of the contralateral pelvic limb whilst the affected limb is balancing on the cushion. This will increase the stabilising muscle strength in the limb and also further challenge his ability to balance. Hold each limb lift for 5 seconds and repeat five times.

   Wobble boards can also be used to challenge balance and improve strength. The patient walks onto the board and faces forwards. Start by gently wobbling the board in an anterior/posterior motion. If the patient tolerates this progress to challenge the patient's balance in the medial/lateral motion. Progress this exercise further to target a limb by incorporating limb lifting into the exercise; start by lifting a pelvic limb. This will force the patient to take more weight through the standing limb, thus increasing strength, and challenging balance.

Because a dog takes 60% of his bodyweight through his thoracic limbs this exercise can be further progressed again by lifting the contralateral thoracic limb (diagonal limb lifting), forcing the patient to shift his weight back onto the pelvic limb to increase strength and balance. Hold each limb lift for 5 seconds and repeat five times.

The owner can be taught how to carry out the limb-lifting exercises at home. The owner could also have the patient walk in figures-of-eight or in circles to challenge balance. Start with wide figures-of-eight and circles, and then progress by making them smaller.

2 *Stamina and cardiovascular (CV) fitness*: will start to improve as the patient is allowed more lead exercise at this stage. Hydrotherapy can be useful in the late stages of rehabilitation as the speed of the belt can be increased to a fast walking pace or gentle trot; this will also improve joint ROM as the patient will take longer strides and improve extensor muscle strength as he propels himself forwards. The level of the water can also be adjusted to give a strengthening effect. The greatest resistance of the water is at the surface level so this level should correspond with the level of the muscle groups you are aiming to strengthen. Resistance can be added by using the UWT water jets; this will further increase strengthening. The work time can also be increased, and the rest time decreased to increase stamina and CV fitness.

Musculoskeletal presenting conditions

The coxofemoral joint

Common conditions associated with the coxofemoral joint, or hip joint as it is often referred to, include:

- Hip dysplasia.
- Legg–Calvé–Perthes disease.
- Fractures.
- Luxations.

The coxofemoral joint is stabilised by the:

- Teres ligament.
- Joint capsule.
- Dorsal acetabular rim.
- Surrounding muscles.

Hip dysplasia (HD)

Hip dysplasia is described as an abnormal development of the coxofemoral joint characterised by subluxation or complete luxation of the femoral head from the acetabulum in young animals (<1 year old) leading to degenerative joint disease in later life.

HD is thought to be a multifactorial disease process. The *primary* cause is thought to be hereditary, and the incidence of HD is highest in large breeds of dogs including Labradors and German shepherd dogs. *Environmental* factors cited include rapid weight gain, rapid growth and over-exercise.

Hip dysplasia is also seen in humans. However, this is not considered a hereditary condition and is not screened for. The primary cause in humans relates to the size (large) and presentation of the foetus. The incidence is highest in large female babies who develop in a confined space with the hip joint flexed and rotated. All babies are assessed for excessive hip laxity shortly after birth. If hip dysplasia is confirmed the baby is fitted with a special hip brace, which is worn for most of the day for a period of months to correct the hip deformity.

However, the disease process of HD in animals is described as:

- Slackening of coxofemoral joint ligaments.
- Subluxation of the femoral head from the acetabulum.
- Destruction of cartilage surfaces.
- A change in shape of joint surface, the femoral head becomes flattened, and the acetabulum becomes shallow.

Secondary osteoarthritis develops resulting in new bone growth at the destroyed cartilage sites, and the formation of fibrous tissue within the joint space as an attempt to provide joint stability.

History

1 Joint instability/wobbly pelvic limb gait pattern.
2 Pain, especially on end-of-range hip extension, and later abduction.
3 Muscle atrophy, especially in gluteals.
4 Difficulty rising, especially after lying for a long period of time, which is common in the morning, or following exercise.
5 Exercise intolerance or reduced levels of exercise.

Physical examination

1 Increased hip laxity caused by weakened ligaments and sub/luxation of the hip joint.
2 Reduced ROM in the hip joint, caused by remodelling of the joint surfaces and associated joint fibrosis.
3 Poor musculature; the animal will be reluctant to weight-bear through the affected limb and will attempt to shift weight onto other limbs, often most evident in stance.

Hip dysplasia – general management

Dietary management: control weight gain especially in immature animals that are still growing. Immature joints have a higher degree of mobility; increased weight gain will place further stress on these developing joints.

Exercise management: again in immature animals that are still growing excessive uncontrolled exercise can place the developing hip joint under increased stress, which may lead to an abnormally developing joint.

Pain control: short-term use of 1–3 weeks' analgesia and strict rest may be prescribed by a veterinary surgeon if indicated.

Nutraceuticals: these may be considered as an adjunct to therapy. The aim of these natural products is to protect the cartilage surfaces and prevent the formation of new bone forming at these sites. Since the changes in cartilage occur early in the disease process the use of nutraceuticals should commence at an early stage also.

Chondroprotectants and nutraceuticals are compounds that are proposed to have a positive effect on the health and metabolism of chondrocytes and synoviocytes (Beal, 2004).

Chondroprotective agents have three main effects:

1. To support or enhance metabolism of chondrocytes and synoviocytes (anabolic).
2. To inhibit degradative enzymes in the synovial fluid and cartilage matrix (catabolic).
3. To inhibit formation of thrombi in the small blood vessels supplying the joint (antithrombotic) (Beal, 2004).

A combination of glucosamine hydrochloride, chondroitin sulphate, manganese and ascorbate is a commonly used nutraceutical in osteoarthritic small animals (Hulse, 1998). The use of these nutritional supplements is supported by clinical studies investigating the treatment of osteoarthritis (Leeb et al., 2000).

Cosequin® has also been found to suppress the anti-inflammatory effects of acute synovitis and immune-mediated arthritis (Beren et al., 2001; Canapp et al., 1999).

Hip dysplasia – conservative versus invasive surgery

The surgical options for hip dysplasia include total hip replacement (THR) or femoral head and neck excision (FHNE) (Figure 1.3). However, when choosing between conservative therapy and surgery, one should take into account the animal's age and current level of activity. The aim of the rehabilitation programme should be to return the animal to its highest level of function. A case study of a conservative rehabilitation programme illustrates a typical approach taken with a 12-month-old dog.

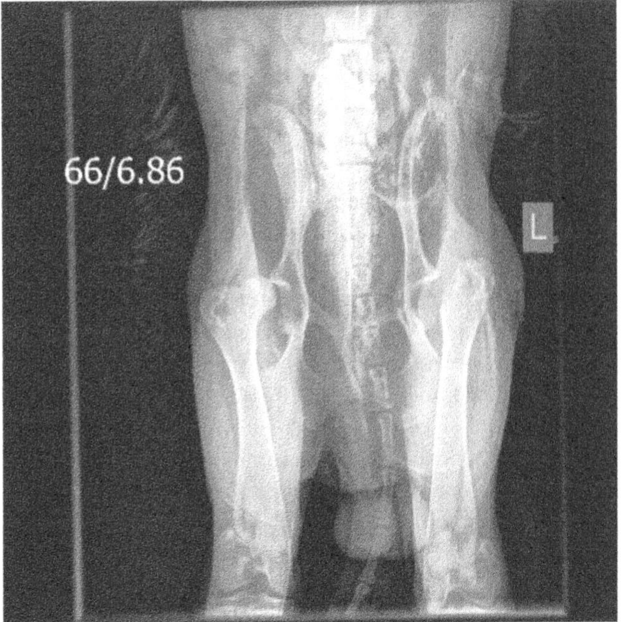

Figure 1.3 Severe hip dysplasia with a left femoral head and neck excision.

CASE STUDY: A PHYSIOTHERAPY REHABILITATION PROGRAMME (CONSERVATIVE) FOR HIP DYSPLASIA

Introduction

'Harvey' is a 12-month-old, male, entire Labrador retriever.

Presenting condition (PC): He presented to the referring veterinary surgeon because he was stiff to rise, but the stiffness eased relatively quickly when the dog walked around for a few minutes.

Past medical history (*PMH*): Nil of note. Harvey is up to date with routine vaccinations and worming. His body weight is optimal.

Drug history (*DH*): A 10-day course of a non-steroidal anti-inflammatory drug (NSAID) was prescribed by the veterinary surgeon to treat his flare-up of pain, and he is on glucosamine and chondroitin supplement long term.

Social history (*SH*): Harvey enjoys walks and chasing balls. He has four walks a day, two longer off-lead walks of one hour duration, playing with other dogs and chasing balls. Two shorter lead walks of approximately 10 minutes. He has free access to a garden. He has stairs in the house but doesn't need to go upstairs. He does not live with any other animals.

Referral details: The referring veterinary surgeon diagnosed Harvey with hip dysplasia; the right pelvic limb was found to be more affected than the left pelvic limb.

Physiotherapy assessment

- *Gait*: 2/5 lame right pelvic limb, with reduced hip extension and slight hip internal rotation.
- *Posture*: Shifts weight from right pelvic limb to left pelvic limb in stance.
- *PROM*: Reduced hip extension and abduction, right more affected than left pelvic limb. Pain is evident on passive hip extension, at end of range.
- *Muscle mass*: Reduced bulk especially hamstrings and gluteals; right more affected than left pelvic limb; right pelvic limb 32 cm, left pelvic limb 34 cm.
- *Muscle length*: Slightly tight hamstrings bilateral.
- *Static weight-bearing percent on pelvic limbs*: Right pelvic limb 42%, left pelvic limb 58%.
- *Pain score*: 2/4 on manipulation of coxofemoral joint.

Problem list

1 Coxofemoral joint pain.
2 Reduced coxofemoral joint ROM (hip extension).
3 Reduced muscle length (hamstrings).
4 Reduced muscle mass right pelvic limb.
5 Altered gait pattern with reduced pelvic limb function.

Goals

1 Reduce pain (2–6 weeks).
2 Improve hip joint ROM (6 weeks).

3 Improve muscle length (6 weeks).
4 Improve muscle mass and strength (6–12 weeks).
5 Gait re-education (6–12 weeks).

Treatment

Therapeutic laser

Apply bilateral laser treatment to the hips, to reduce pain; the power and time (duration) of treatment will depend on the patient's skin colour, bodyweight and stage of condition (acute or chronic).

PROM exercises

To maintain joint ROM at the hip, stifle and tarsus joints. All joints are flexed, and then extended. Rotation of the limb is avoided, with one hand supporting at the medial stifle joint. Note that the limb is not gripped and no pulling of the limb occurs; the distal hand pushes the limb into flexion, then the proximal hand, which is medial and anterior to the stifle joint, pushes the limb into extension.

Three sets of 10 PROM repetitions are performed on each pelvic limb; there is no hold at the end of full flexion or extension so one repetition of pelvic limb PROM should not take more than one to two seconds. Three sets of 10 repetitions should be completed in 30–60 seconds if the patient is compliant.

Passive stretches

Hip flexors, hamstrings and adductors are stretched passively. Again avoid any rotation of the joints of the pelvic limb and support the distal limb. Each stretch should be taken into resistance and held for 15 seconds and repeated three times. Stretching should not be painful for the patient. If the patient is very tense gentle warm-up exercises may assist with stretching, or warming the muscles with heat packs pre-stretching may be beneficial. With hip dysplasia, extension and abduction are usually the most uncomfortable movements for the patient, so be aware that full hip extension and abduction may not be possible if the patient has developed secondary osteoarthritic changes around the hip joint.

Active exercises

Weaving cones – begin by placing the cones approximately the length of the dog's body apart. As he progresses the distance between the cones can be narrowed and more cones may be added. Weaving exercises will encourage the patient to transfer weight onto the affected limb, and will also strengthen adductor and abductor muscles around the hip joint.

Cavaletti poles – aim to place the poles to correspond with the dog's normal stride length to begin with. Start with the poles positioned at an achievable height. As the patient progresses the arrangement of poles can be adjusted to increase limb flexion and joint ROM.

Stairs – are a functional activity and challenge strength and ROM in the pelvic limbs as the patient pushes off to ascend the stair. Balance and weight-bearing through the thoracic limbs are challenged as the patient descends the stairs. Bunnyhopping up the stairs may be seen in animals with reduced ROM or strength in the pelvic limbs; however, bunnyhopping on stairs may be *normal* for small dogs.

Wobble board – this equipment should be introduced gradually to ensure patient compliance. With the patient positioned with all four limbs on the board passively rock the board left and right to challenge the patient's right or left side limbs. Alternatively the patient may be positioned to challenge thoracic or pelvic limbs by rocking the board forwards and backwards. This exercise will improve stability around the hip joint; as the patient resists the movement of the board his stabilising and postural muscles will be activated.

Underwater treadmill (UWT) – begin with short-duration sessions and use the buoyancy effect of the water to reduce the load and concussive forces passing through the joints of the limbs. If the patient has severe osteoarthritis secondary to hip dysplasia he will find exercising in the UWT comfortable. The temperature of the water, level of the water and speed of the treadmill belt can all be controlled.

Progression

Wobble board: This exercise can be progressed by incorporating limb lifting (Figure 1.4).

UWT: Increasing the duration of exercising in the treadmill will improve stamina. Increasing the speed of the belt will improve joint ROM and stride length. The water level can be lowered to reduce the buoyancy effect of the water and improve strengthening. Further strengthening can be achieved by using resistance from the water jets.

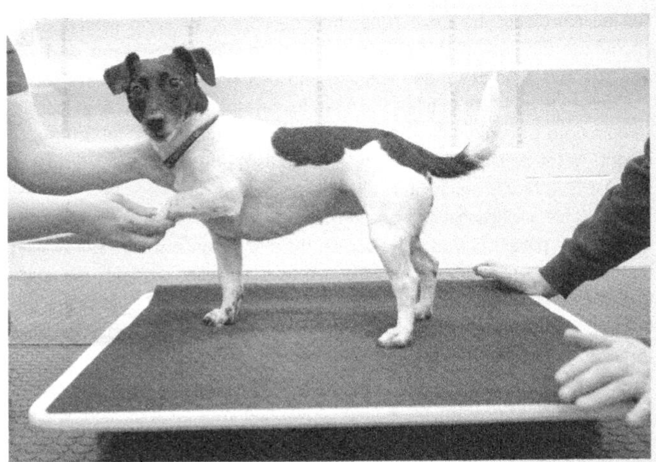

Figure 1.4 A patient balancing on a wobble board. The left thoracic limb is lifted to target strengthening and stability in the right thoracic limb.

Evaluation

It is important to evaluate treatment to ensure it is effective. Once a patient has achieved his short-term goals progress him on to improve joint ROM and muscle length in the mid-phase rehabilitation programme, then finally in the late phase of rehabilitation progress him again to improve strength and muscle mass, to rehabilitate him back to his highest level of function.

Outcome measures

Baseline measures should be taken at the time of the first assessment. Assuming the patient is attending on a weekly basis re-measure outcomes at 6 and 12 weeks.

Joint ROM – of the coxofemoral joint using a goniometer should be taken at the initial assessment. Measure and record passive hip extension, abduction and flexion.

Muscle mass – can be measured using a tape measure. Aim to measure around the muscle belly of the hamstrings/quadriceps; this will approximately be at the level of the mid-femur. As the patient begins to build muscle mass and strength this will show with a increase in muscle circumference. It is good practice to take three measures, and then use the average from these readings as the final measure.

Gait – video the patient's gait pattern at the initial assessment. This can then be compared to later videos to demonstrate positive changes in gait pattern. The lameness score can also be assessed from the videos.

Function – measure weight-bearing through the affected limb and the contralateral limb for comparison of limb function at the time of assessment it will be a useful measurement to re-test as the animal progresses. Normal bathroom weighing scales have been shown to be a valid measuring tool to assess weight-bearing in dogs.

Pain – subjectively the owner may provide feedback such as the dog's ability to walk further, or a willingness to play with other dogs and toys without any signs of increased lameness or difficulty rising. The owner may also feedback a decrease in the patient's analgesic requirement. Pain score measures should be repeated at 6 and 12 weeks and compared with baseline to evaluate the effectiveness of treatment.

Stifle joint

The canine stifle is made up of bones that form joints, which are supported by ligaments and menisci.

Anatomy

Bones

- Femur.
- Tibia.
- Patella.
- Fabellae.
- Popliteal sesamoid.

Joints

- Femoral-tibial.
- Patella-femoral.

Ligaments

- Cranial cruciate ligament – stabilises the tibia relative to the femur to prevent hyperextension and also internal rotation of the tibia.
- Caudal cruciate ligament – stabilises the tibia to prevent caudal displacement relative to the femur.
- Medial and lateral collateral ligaments – prevent valgus and varus movement of the stifle joint.

Menisci

- Medial.
- Lateral.

Cruciate ligament injury

Cruciate injury is a relatively common condition in small animals. It is typically seen in young active dogs. Presentation maybe seen as an acute, chronic or a partial tear.

Aetiology

Canine cruciate ligament (CCL) rupture may be acute and related to trauma, and seen in any breed. Chronic injury occurs over a period of time and may be multifactorial in nature. Obesity and muscle imbalances may contribute to chronic cruciate injury. Partial tears can cause pain and inflammation; if the tear is minor it may settle with rest and conservative treatment. However, major partial tears may require a more invasive approach (surgery) (Figure 1.5).

It may be worth noting that not all humans or indeed animals undergo surgical procedures to stabilise a ruptured cruciate ligament. Over time capsular fibrosis occurs and this scar tissue stabilises the joint to some degree. However, a trade-off may be some loss of ROM in the stifle, but the limb will be functional. If the patient goes on to develop a meniscal injury this will require surgical intervention as

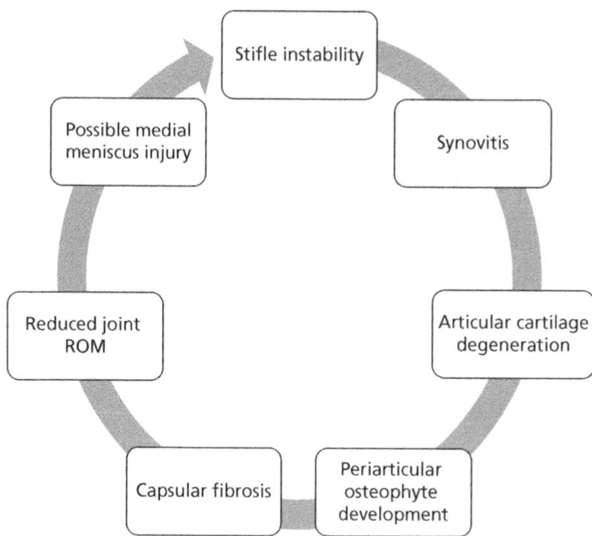

Figure 1.5 Sequence of cranial cruciate ligament disease events.

pain will be present when the animal flexes and loads the joint, resulting in chronic lameness. Secondary osteoarthritis of the stifle joint will occur as a consequence of CCL injury.

Clinical signs

- Lameness – non-weight bearing if acute, subtle lameness associated with exercise in early partial tears.
- Joint effusion – seen in the acute stage, and is part of the normal injury inflammatory process.
- Fibrosis – (medial buttress), palpate medial aspect of stifle joint and compare with the contralateral stifle.

- Muscle atrophy – (indicates its not an acute injury).
- Decreased ROM of the affected stifle.
- Crepitus or meniscal clicking of the stifle during passive flexion and extension may be evident.

Conservative treatment

- Rest.
- Non-steroidal anti-inflammatory drugs (NSAIDs) for 6 weeks.
- Weight reduction (if appropriate).
- Controlled exercise to strengthen the hamstring muscle group to stabilise the tibia and prevent *forward draw* of the tibia.

Surgical treatment

Extracapsular:

- Lateral fabellar suture.

Intracapsular:

- Over-the-top technique (OTT).
- Tibial plateau levelling osteotomy (TPLO).
- Tibial tuberosity advancement (TTA).
- Tibial wedge osteotomy (TWO).
- Triple tibial osteotomy (TTO).

Tibial osteotomies all aim to eliminate cranial tibial thrust, and provide long-term stability of the stifle joint. Long-term studies are required to provide evidence of each technique's effectiveness.

Complications

- Infection.
- Implant failure.
- Late meniscal injury.
- Persistent lameness.
- Osteoarthritis.
- Rupture of contralateral cruciate ligament.

CASE STUDY: A PHYSIOTHERAPY REHABILITATION PROGRAMME FOR CANINE CRUCIATE LIGAMENT RUPTURE (CONSERVATIVE)

History

Buster is a 12-year-old neutered Labrador. He has a right stifle cranial cruciate ligament rupture and is being referred for physiotherapy. He is overweight at 40 kg, and is currently on a calorie-restricted diet.

Assessment

1. Right stifle pain on manipulation 2/4 (0–4 scale).
2. PROM: resents end-of-range flexion and extension of right stifle, mild joint effusion and thickening of stifle joint medially. (Right flexion 40°, right extension 155°; left flexion 45°, left extension 160°).
3. Muscle length: tight right hamstrings.
4. Muscle mass: reduced global bulk right pelvic limb (right circumference 26 cm, left 29 cm).
5. Weight-bearing: shifts weight in stance onto contralateral pelvic limb (right 40%, left 60%).
6. Gait: toe touching lame right pelvic limb (videoed).

Problem list

1. Right stifle pain.
2. Reduced ROM right stifle.
3. Reduced muscle length right hamstrings.
4. Reduced muscle mass right pelvic limb.
5. Reduced right pelvic limb function.
6. Abnormal gait pattern.

Goals

1. Reduce pain (2–6 weeks).
2. Improve right stifle ROM (6 weeks).
3. Improve hamstring length right pelvic limb (6 weeks).
4. Improve strength right pelvic limb (6–12 weeks).
5. Improve right pelvic limb weight-bearing (6–12 weeks).
6. Gait re-education (6–12 weeks).

Passive exercises

PROM: An exercise to maintain joint ROM; three sets of 10 repetitions are recommended. The three major joints in the pelvic limb are flexed together and then extended; take care to avoid any rotation of the joints especially the stifle. With the patient lying in left lateral recumbency use one hand to support the stifle joint medially; the other hand is placed below the calcaneus and pushes all the joints into flexion; the first hand will push from the distal femur to bring the joints into extension. *N.B. No pulling or harsh gripping of the tissues occurs. Do not force full stifle flexion/extension in the early stage.*

Stretches: Gentle progressive stretches of hamstring muscle groups; three stretches into resistance held for 15 seconds is recommended. If the patient has been lame for some time the hip flexor muscle group may also be tight: three stretches into resistance held for 15 seconds is recommended. *N.B. Stretching should not be painful for the animal, but ensure the stretch is into resistance to obtain effective treatment – the aim of the stretches is to increase muscle length.*

Laser therapy: To reduce pain and inflammation of the stifle joint.

Active exercises

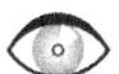
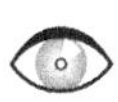

Weaving cones: To encourage weight transfer onto the affected limb, and to encourage abduction and adduction of the affected limb (Video 1.1).

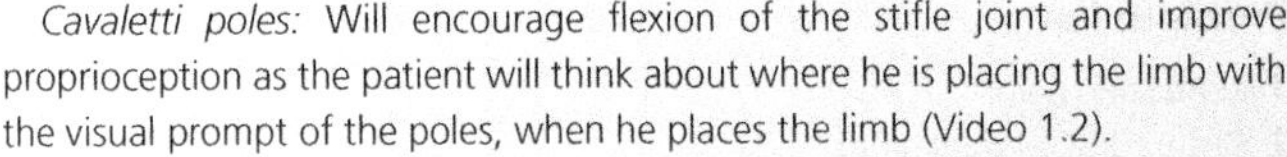
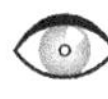

Cavaletti poles: Will encourage flexion of the stifle joint and improve proprioception as the patient will think about where he is placing the limb with the visual prompt of the poles, when he places the limb (Video 1.2).

Stairs: This is a functional activity and so should be practised in a controlled environment. The patient will require strength in the pelvic limbs to ascend the stairs; balance and proprioception will be challenged as the patient descends the stairs; keep in close to the patient so that if he loses balance on the stairs you will be able to support him.

VIDEO 1.1

Weaving cones. The video shows a patient being led through weaving cones to encourage limb weight transfer and abduction and adduction of the limbs. This active exercise also encourages lateral spinal flexion.

VIDEO 1.2

Cavalleti poles. The video shows a patient being led over equally spaced cavaletti poles. This active exercise improves joint ROM as the patient flexes his limbs to clear the pole. As the patient progresses the height of the poles can be increased. This exercise also challenges and therefore improves proprioception because the patient will use the visual prompt of the poles to think about how high he will need to flex his limb and also where he will place his limb. This exercise can be progressed by increasing the height of the poles, or arranging the poles alternately high then low.

Wobble cushions: This exercise is used to strengthen the muscles to stabilise the affected limb; it will also challenge and therefore improve balance. Place the wobble cushion under the affected limb and nudge the patient at the contralateral limb so that he is taking weight on an unstable surface through the affected limb(Figure 1.6). Progress this exercise by incorporating limb lifting of the unaffected pelvic limb while the patient is weight-bearing through the affected limb on the wobble cushion (Figure 1.7). Hold the unaffected limb for 5 seconds; let the patient rest then repeat for a total of five repetitions. *N.B. Support the patient under the abdomen with your arm as necessary until he builds confidence and strength with this exercise.*

Wobble board: Once the patient has mastered the wobble cushion progress to the wobble board; keep the session time on the wobble board short to begin with until the patient becomes accustomed to the exercise. The patient stands with all four limbs on the wobble board. By passively rocking the board forwards the patient will be taking weight through the thoracic limbs, and when rocked backwards the patient will be taking weight through the pelvic limbs. If the patient changes direction the left and right side limbs can be challenged. This exercise will improve strength and stability in the limbs, and improve general core strength and stability. The exercise can be progressed by incorporating limb lifting; lifting the unaffected pelvic limb will strengthen and stabilise the affected pelvic limb. To further change the patient progress by lifting the contralateral thoracic limb.

N.B. Support the patient under the abdomen with your arm as necessary until he builds confidence and strength with this exercise.

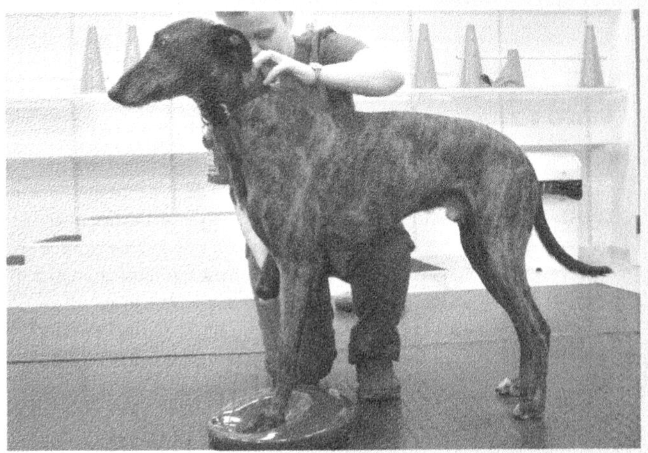

Figure 1.6 A patient's left thoracic limb on the wobble cushion, with the right thoracic limb lifted. This unstable surface will challenge and improve conscious proprioception in the left thoracic limb. This exercise also has a strengthening/stabilising effect on the limb.

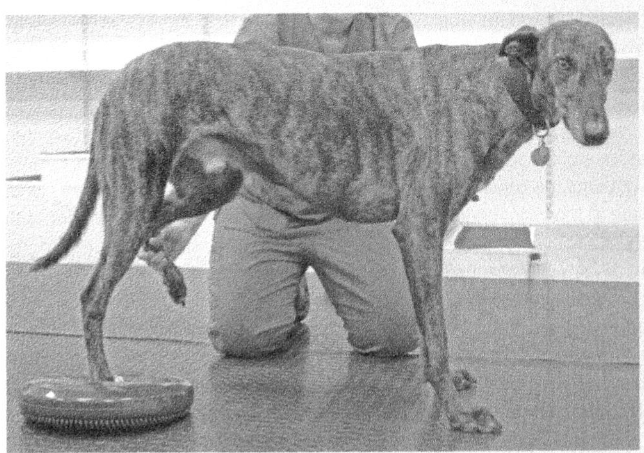

Figure 1.7 A patient weight-bearing and balancing on a wobble cushion. The left pelvic limb is lifted to further strengthen and stabilise the right pelvic limb.

Hydrotherapy: Walking in an UWT will increase limb ROM, and improve functional ability as the warmth of the water and buoyancy effect will provide the patient with a comfortable environment to exercise in with reduced concussive forces passing through the limbs. Begin with short sessions and provide plenty of rest breaks. Initially, set the treadmill belt slower than the patient's normal gait speed to ensure he is using the limb functionally and weight-bearing through the affected limb.

As the patient progresses use the water to provide strengthening rather than buoyancy so the patient has to push through the water to build muscle strength. The surface level of the water is where most resistance is found so set the water level to mid-femur to improve muscle strengthening. Increasing the speed of the treadmill belt will encourage the patient to take longer strides, which will increase ROM and encourage extensor muscle activity and therefore strength. Using water jets to provide resistance will also further strengthen the patient. Increasing the exercise time and reducing the rest time will improve cardiovascular fitness and stamina.

Rehabilitation following surgical repair of cranial cruciate ligament rupture

CCL rupture treated by surgical repair would tend to follow a similar rehabilitation programme (Figures 1.8 and 1.9). Ensure you are familiar with the type of CCL repair the patient has undergone – that is, extracapsular lateral suture repair or open reduction internal fixation (ORIF) osteotomy stabilisation. Generally a patient would be referred following suture removal and a satisfactory check-up by the veterinary surgeon. (Alternatively the surgeon may wait until 6 weeks postoperatively to refer the patient for physiotherapy.)

In the early phase (0–2 weeks postoperatively) focus on gentle ROM exercises to maintain joint ROM. Stretches of the hip flexors, hamstrings and adductors will maintain muscle length. Laser therapy can be used to reduce pain and inflammation, as indicated. The patient may be toe touch or PWB; use *The Soft Quick Lift*™ sling to

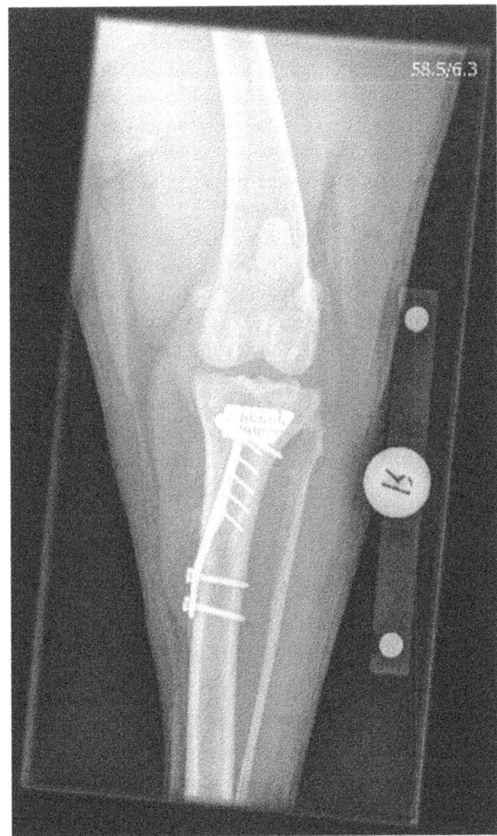

Figure 1.8 A right cranio-caudal postoperative tibial tuberosity advancement.

support the patient and to assist him with balance. Short, gentle, controlled lead exercise with sling support for 5 minutes four times daily is recommended in the early phase. When using a sling support the owner should take up a position at the hip on the same side as the

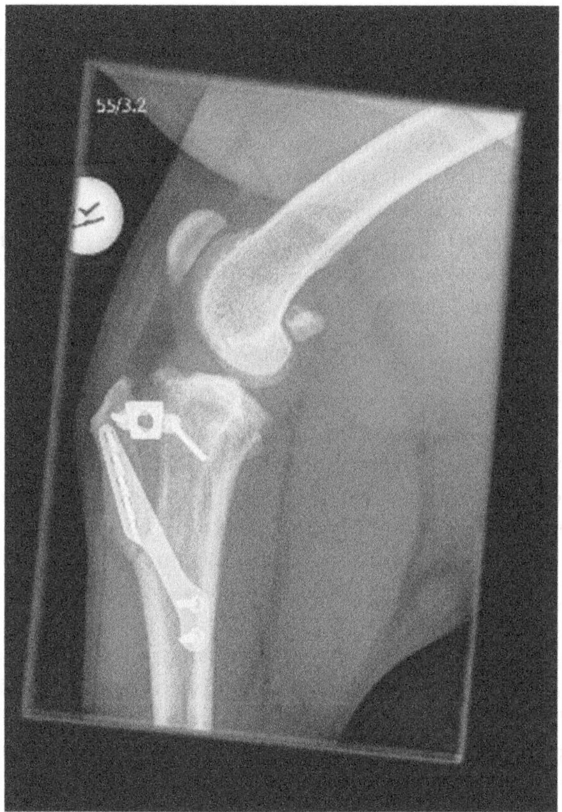

Figure 1.9 A right lateral postoperative tibial tuberosity advancement.

unaffected limb so they can gently transfer the patient's bodyweight onto the unaffected limb, but whilst taking some bodyweight so as not to overload the unaffected limb.

In the mid-phase (2–6 weeks postoperatively), continue with the PROM exercises, stretches and laser therapy from the early phase, and begin to introduce active assisted exercises (active assisted exercises incorporate the use of a sling to prevent the patient from losing balance, and also to prevent him taking excessive weight through the affected limb). Weaving exercises, cavaletti pole work and hydrotherapy using a UWT to encourage functional use of the limb can all begin at this stage. The patient will not require the use of a sling in hydrotherapy because the buoyancy of the water will support the patient's balance and reduce bodyweight and concussive forces passing through the limbs. However, a member of staff should also be in the water with the patient for safety and reassurance should he panic, and to support him with the sling into and out of the water treadmill.

In the late phase (6–12 weeks) the patient should have regained full ROM of the joint and normal muscle length. He should also have started to increase weight-bearing through the limb and therefore have improved strength and function in the limb. He may now only be dependent on the sling when his strength, balance and proprioception are challenged, such as on stairs, which can be introduced to the patient at this stage in a controlled environment. The number of weaving cones and height of cavaletti poles can also be increased at this stage.

Towards the end of the late phase introduce balance changes with wobble cushions, progress balance, and improve limb stability and strength by incorporating limb lifting into the exercise. This exercise can be progressed by introducing the wobble board, which challenges balance in all limbs, and in four planes of movement. The wobble board also improves core stability, limb strength and stability.

Hydrotherapy using a UWT is a functional way for the patient to increase ROM, strength and improve CV fitness. The water can be used to provide resistance and further resistance can be added by using water jets. The speed of the belt can be increased to encourage longer strides to improve ROM of the joints; rest breaks can be reduced and time spent exercising in the UWT increased to improve CV fitness.

Following a satisfactory 12-week check from the veterinary surgeon the owner can commence with short periods of off-lead exercise in an enclosed space.

Evaluation of rehabilitation

Aim to evaluate the patient's progress at regular intervals. Measure baseline data at assessment, and re-measure at 6 and 12 weeks to evaluate the effectiveness of treatment, and to guide progression of the rehabilitation programme.

- Assess and score pain on manipulation of the limb, and from the owner's feedback.
- Measure joint ROM using a goniometer.
- Measure the circumference of muscle mass around the muscle belly; compare with the contralateral limb measures.
- Measure weight-bearing through the limb using bathroom scales, or a pressure-sensitive mat.
- Video gait pattern, and score lameness (0–5 scale).

Obtaining optimal hamstring length and strength is important; the hamstring muscle group is made up of:

- Biceps femoris.
- Semitendinosus.
- Semimembranosus.

This group of muscles insert on the tibia, and have an important role in stabilising the tibia and preventing the characteristic *forward-draw* of the tibia over the femur seen in patients with deficient cranial cruciate ligament function.

The reason the hamstrings become weak is related to reduced weight-bearing on the affected limb. Progressive stretches of the hamstring muscle group will maintain optimal muscle length.

Scar tissue will form around the affected stifle joint. This is the body's natural way of stabilising the joint. Excessive scar tissue and thickened of the joint capsule will lead to reduced ROM at this joint. Secondary osteoarthritis will also lead to reduced joint ROM, and pain. Excessive scar tissue may be reduced by laser therapy and PROM exercises to maintain functional ROM of the affected joint.

Meniscal tears are a relatively common finding associated with cruciate disease, and will often require surgical intervention. The medial meniscus is most often affected as relatively more weight passes through the medial meniscus when the animal ambulates.

Bilateral cruciate disease may also become evident. This may be related to the extra strain placed on the contralateral pelvic limb.

The patient may also develop changes in the lumbar spine related to abnormal gait pattern and uneven loading through the limbs. This may be seen as muscle tension over the lumbar spine with associated trigger points and lumber spine stiffness on palpation.

Patella luxation

The patella is a sesamiod bone located within the patella ligament. Luxation occurs when the patella rides outside the femoral groove when the stifle is flexed. It can be classified as medial or lateral; medial luxation is most common.

Each time the patella luxates the associated cartilage is at risk of damage, resulting in inflammation and leading to secondary osteoarthritis and pain.

Aetiology

- It can be traumatic (rare).
- It often relates to a shallow femoral groove.
- Muscle imbalance and poor limb alignment may result in patella luxation.
- Or it may be multifactorial in nature.

Incidence

- Often found in small dogs (poodle, Yorkshire terrier, Chihuahua).
- Presentation may be bilateral.

Clinical signs

- Lameness – intermittent or continuous.
- Pain – most evident in acute luxation.
- Bilateral medial patella luxations may have a *bow-legged* conformation.
- Bilateral patella luxations may have a *knock-kneed* conformation.

Diagnosis

- Palpation of the stifle.
- Plain radiographs.
- Computed tomography (CT).

Surgical treatment

Surgical correction involves reconstruction of the soft tissues associated with the patella and deepening of the femoral groove to correct tracking of the patella tendon (Table 1.3). If the luxation is medial the groove can be deepened on the lateral side.

Transposing the tibial crest may be performed to realign the quadriceps and the patella tendon.

The surgery is more challenging if the luxating patella is associated with angulation of the long bones.

Table 1.3 Patella luxation grades.

Grade	Description
I	Patella can be manipulated out of groove, but spontaneously returns to its normal position
II	Patella occasionally moves out of the groove, but can easily be manipulated back in to place
III	Patella moves out of the groove frequently, but can be manipulated back in to place
IV	Patella moves out of the groove persistently and cannot be replaced

Complications

- Reluxation.
- Infection.
- Implant failure.
- Persistent lameness.
- Osteoarthritis.
- Contra-lateral limb affected.

CASE STUDY: PHYSIOTHERAPY REHABILITATION PROGRAMME FOR A LUXATING PATELLA (SURGICAL)

History

Molly is a 2-year-old, female Maltese terrier. She has been referred for physiotherapy following surgery 6 weeks ago to treat a left pelvic limb (PL) luxating patella.

Physiotherapy assessment

- *Gait:* ambulatory, reduced weight-bearing through the left PL, and a reduced stance phase.
- *Lameness score:* intermittently carries limb, lame in trot, score 4/5 (0–5 scale).
- *Posture:* shifts weight from left to right PL in stance.
- *Pain score:* signs of moderate pain during palpation 2/4 (0–4 scale).
- *Joint ROM:* resents left stifle end-of-range (EoR) flexion/extension.
- *Muscle length:* tight in hip flexors, weak in hamstrings.
- *Muscle mass:* reduced bulk left PL; 1.5 cm difference compared to right PL.
- *Secondary complications:* nil obvious at this stage.

Problem list

1. Altered gait pattern.
2. Pain.
3. Reduced joint ROM.
4. Muscle imbalance.
5. Reduced strength/muscle mass.

Goals

1 Gait re-education.
2 Reduce pain.
3 Improve joint ROM.
4 Improve muscle imbalance.
5 Improve strength/muscle mass.

Physiotherapy out patient treatment plan

Early phase (0–2 weeks)

- Control pain and reduce swelling using cold therapy, or laser.
- Improve stifle and patella femoral joint ROM, using gentle PROM exercises.
- Short controlled lead walking 4 × 5 minutes a day.

Mid-phase (2–6 weeks)

- Continue laser therapy for pain control, and to control scar tissue.
- Continue PROM exercises and stretches.
- Begin proprioceptive exercises using cavaletti poles.
- Use weaving cones to encourage weight transfer onto the affected limb.
- Begin strengthening exercises using the UWT.
- Increase lead walks to 4 × 10 minutes a day.

Late phase (6–12 weeks)

- Continue laser, PROM exercises, begin soft tissue release techniques (STR), to ensure smooth patella mobility.
- Continue with cavaletti pole and weaving cone work.
- Challenge balance and proprioception using a wobble cushion and incorporate limb lifting to improve strength and stability.
- Introduce stair work, encourage the owner to introduce gentle gradients into the patient's lead walks, which should increase to 4 × 15 minutes a day.
- Progress hydrotherapy by increasing the time the patient spends working in the treadmill and reduce the water level to reduce buoyancy so the water is used to provide resistance.

Evaluation

Outcome baseline measures obtained at initial assessment should be repeated at 6 and 12 weeks to evaluate the rehabilitation programme and to guide progression.

Progression

Following a satisfactory check with the veterinary surgeon introduce work on the wobble board and incorporate limb lifting into the rehabilitation programme. Progress hydrotherapy by increasing the speed of the belt and use extra resistance from the water jets. The owner can allow the patient to have short periods of off-lead exercise in a controlled confined space.

Discharge

The patient would normally be discharged from physiotherapy at around 12 weeks assuming she has achieved the goals defined by the physiotherapy problem list. If the patient has not progressed as expected, she may require further physiotherapy or referral back to her own veterinary surgeon for further investigation.

Limb amputation

Most small animals have the ability to ambulate on three limbs; they can adapt well to the change, and maintain a good quality of life. Amputation may be performed as a salvage procedure following extreme trauma to a limb, or it may be an elective procedure; for example, in the case of bone neoplasia the limb may be amputated.

An accurate medical history for the animal must be taken to ensure the rehabilitation programme is suitable for the individual animal. If the animal has neoplasia with chest metastasis he may have reduced stamina so the physiotherapy programme needs to reflect this and be adapted to meet the animal's and owner's needs.

Consideration must be given to the loading on the other limbs following amputation. This is especially important should the animal be overweight; if this is the case the animal should also be on a calorie-controlled diet. If a thoracic limb has been amputated the contralateral forelimb will have an increased load through the joints. Keep in mind that dogs take 60% of their bodyweight through their thoracic limbs. If a pelvic limb has been amputated the animal may learn to distribute its weight diagonally onto the contralateral thoracic limb.

Ideally the animal would not be overweight, have good ROM in all joints in the remaining three limbs, have no concurrent joint disease such as osteoarthritis, and good muscle mass and strength in the remaining three limbs.

However, the animal will still be at risk of secondary complications due to the change in weight-bearing through the limbs. Rotation of the spinal column towards the side of the amputation often occurs, especially if the animal has poor balance. This can lead to permanent changes and stiffness in the skeletal spine and associated muscle imbalances resulting in chronic pain.

It is important to educate the owner on lifestyle changes for the animal following amputation. If the dog previously jumped in and out of the car this may now be impossible or inappropriate for the animal. The dog may previously been taken on very long daily walks. The energy requirement for an amputee to walk is much greater than for its quadrupedal counterpart, and this should be taken into consideration. The animal may find shorter, gentler walks most enjoyable following amputation.

Until recently in veterinary practice it has been normal procedure to amputate the whole of the limb. Recent developments in veterinary practice include fitting animals with prosthetic weight-bearing devices. This type of surgery in animals is still in its early stages and is by no means a routine elective procedure.

Physiotherapy rehabilitation programme post limb amputation

Early phase (0–2 weeks)

- Control pain and encourage wound healing with laser therapy.
- Reduce swelling at the surgical site using cold therapy.
- Reduce compensatory muscle soreness using massage, heat therapy and STR techniques.
- Reduce load on adjacent hind limb, use The Soft Quick Lift™ sling to support the patient and to assist him with maintaining his balance.

Mid-phase (2–4 weeks)

- Begin muscle strengthening exercises.
- Introduce proprioceptive and balance exercises.

Late phase (4–6 weeks)

- Begin to introduce functional activities (stairs, getting in and out of car consider using a ramp).
- Improve CV fitness and stamina. If available use a UWT, the water will support the patient, and he may be able to exercise for longer.
- Increase the duration of walks, and reduce the support from the sling if able to.

N.B. Be aware of the additional energy requirement the amputee will face, so pace the rehabilitation programme to the patient's ability levels, and do not allow him to fatigue.

Elbow joint

The elbow consists of three main bones:

- Humerus.
- Radius.
- Ulna.

The articulations of these bones make up the three joints of the elbow:

- Humero-radial.
- Humero-ulnar.
- Proximal radio-ulnar.

The medial and lateral collateral annular ligaments support these joints. The main nerves associated with the thoracic limb are:

- Radial nerve.
- Median nerve.
- Ulnar nerve.

Damage to any of these nerves can occur with luxation of the elbow joint.

Elbow dysplasia

'Elbow dysplasia' is a general term used to describe various developmental abnormalities within the elbow joint. It is a relatively common finding in canines, especially large breeds such as Labradors and Rottweilers. Elbow dysplasia may be classified as:

- Fragmentation of the medial coronoid process (FMCP).
- Osteochondritis dissecans (OCD) of the medial condyle.
- Un-united anconeal process (UAP).
- Un-united medial epicondyle.
- Elbow joint incongruity.

Presentation

- Often young dogs 6–9 months old.
- Thoracic limb lameness – often bilateral.
- Flicking of carpi when walking, elbows often abducted.
- Painful elbow joint on manipulation.
- Reduced ROM in elbow, especially flexion with supination (increases pressure on medial coronoid process resulting in pain).

- Crepitus.
- Muscle atrophy.

Elbow dysplasia – fragmented medial coronoid process (FMCP)

This condition results in possible fragmentation of the medial coronoid and cartilage erosions resulting in elbow pain and instability.

Aetiology

- A form of osteochondrosis (micro fractures).
- Found secondary to elbow incongruity and abnormal loading through the joint.
- A short radius (resulting in increased pressure on medial coronoid process).
- Leads to trochlear notch dysplasia (resulting in increased pressure and pain).

Diagnosis

- Plain radiographs (sometimes not obvious).
- CT.
- Arthroscopy.

Treatment

- Medical management (NSAIDs, rest).
- Arthroscopic removal of osteochondral fragment.
- Debridement of underlying bone and removal of loose cartilage.
- An ulnar osteotomy may be considered in severe cases.

Elbow dysplasia – osteochondritis dissecans (OCD)

Osteochondritis dissecans (OCD) is a failure of endochondral ossification. A tear develops in the cartilage leaving a flap, which leads to pain and inflammation within the joint. The condition is often seen in large and giant breeds of dog; the elbow or other joints (shoulder, stifle) can be affected.

Aetiology

OCD lesions are often found on the medial humeral condyle, seen as a cleft or flap in the cartilage.

Diagnosis

- Plain radiographs (sometimes not obvious).
- CT.
- Arthroscopy.

Treatment

Removal of flap arthroscopically and curetting of underlying bone.

Elbow dysplasia – un-united anconeal process (UAP)

Un-united anconeal process (UAP) occurs when the anconeal process fails to fuse with the olecranon.

Aetiology

- A form of osteochondrosis.
- Found secondary to elbow incongruity and abnormal loading.
- A long radius, results in pressure on humerus and anconeal process, which in turn becomes un-united.
- Leads to trochlear notch dysplasia (resulting in increased pressure and pain).

Diagnosis

- Plain radiographs (usually obvious).
- Do not radiograph before 4–5 months of age as there could be a secondary centre of ossification.

Treatment

- Removal has variable results and can lead to an unstable elbow.
- Ulnar osteotomy, to remove the pressure and allow fusing, is not always successful.
- Lag screw fixation and ulnar osteotomy is technically difficult to achieve but the results are good.

Long-term progression of osteoarthritis is inevitable.

Elbow dysplasia – incongruity

Aetiology

- Unknown.

Diagnosis

- Plain radiographs (difficult as limb position influences interpretation).
- CT is more reliable than radiographs.
- Arthroscopy.

Treatment

Ulnar shortening/lengthening procedures.

Elbow dysplasia – prognosis

- Variable.
- Secondary osteoarthritis inevitable in all cases.
- Outcome improved if cartilage erosions are reduced in extent on arthroscopy.

Incomplete ossification of the humeral condyle (IOHC)

This is a failure of bony union between humeral condyles, predisposing to humeral condylar fractures.

Aetiology

Unknown. *Almost exclusively seen in springer spaniels.*

Treatment

Transcondylar screws if clinically affected.

Elbow trauma

- Traumatic luxation, mainly lateral due to anatomy.
- Fractures of the distal humerus.
- Olecranon fractures.
- Ulnar fractures with radial head luxation.
- Radial fractures.

Traumatic luxation

Clinical signs

- Lameness.
- Increased elbow width.
- Reduced extension.

Diagnosis

Radiographs to confirm.

Treatment

- Closed reduction.
- Open reduction internal fixation (ORIF).
- Ligament repair.

Aftercare

If no ligament damage present:

- Robert Jones dressing for 1 week.

- Two weeks controlled lead exercise.
- (ROM will be reduced).

If ligament damage present:

- Splint for 2 weeks.
- Four weeks' lead-controlled exercise.

Commence passive flexion-extension exercises following support removal.

Fractures of the distal humerus

- Lateral condyle (most common).
- Medial condyle (less common).
- Y-fracture (complex).
- T-fracture (complex).

Fractures of the lower thoracic limb

Fractures of the proximal ulna with luxation of the radial head have a guarded prognosis. Secondary complications of osteoarthritis, reduced elbow motion, nerve damage and reluxation of the radial head are common. The elbow joint is a high motion joint and physiotherapy plays an important role in improving ROM once the fracture has consolidated.

Olecranon fractures usually require open reduction and internal fixation (ORIF); stabilisation of the olecranon needs to be such as to eliminate the pull of the triceps muscle, which inserts on the olecranon.

Proximal fractures of the radius are uncommon. Growth plate fracture may be seen in immature animals. Articular fractures require accurate anatomical reduction to minimise secondary osteoarthritic changes. Comminuted fractures carry a poor prognosis; fracture healing times and weight-bearing through the limb may be prolonged.

Fractures may be managed conservatively using casting/splinting methods versus open reduction internal fixation (ORIF) methods.

CASE STUDY: PHYSIOTHERAPY REHABILITATION PROGRAMME FOR A FRACTURED ELBOW REPAIR

Introduction

Bruno is a 2-year-old, male, entire springer spaniel referred to physiotherapy following a left thoracic limb distal humerus lateral condyle fracture (open reduction internal fixation) repair.

Presenting condition (PC): 5/5 lame on left thoracic limb following road traffic accident (RTA). Radiographs demonstrate left thoracic limb distal humerus lateral condyle fracture.

Past medical history (PMH): nil of note. Bruno is up to date with routine vaccinations and worming.

Drug history (DH): short course of NSAID post-surgery, nil at present.

Social history (SH): Bruno was a working gundog, and the owner would like Bruno to return to work if possible. Previously Bruno was kennelled outside with other working dogs, and again the owner would like him to return to this. The owner drives a 4 × 4 vehicle and Bruno would previously jump in and out of the car.

Bruno is now 6 weeks post-operation, and has been referred for physiotherapy.

Physiotherapy assessment

Gait: 2/5 lame on the left thoracic limb. Abducts affected limb when ambulating and in stance.

Posture: reduced weight-bearing through the left thoracic limb, shifting weight onto right thoracic limb.

Static weight-bearing: left thoracic limb 40%, right thoracic limb 60%.

Joint ROM: reduced end-of-range passive elbow flexion and extension of the left thoracic limb.

Muscle length: tight biceps, rhomboids and pectorals, reduced scapular mobility left thoracic limb.

Muscle mass: reduced bulk triceps, infra and supraspinatus left thoracic limb.

Conscious proprioception (CP): normal left thoracic limb.

Pain score: consider if the patient has a functional lameness following surgical intervention, or if the lameness is due to pain. Inflammation of the joint, discomfort on manipulation and a positive response to analgesia would suggest the patient is in pain. Pain scored 2/4.

Aggravating factors: does exercise increase pain and lameness?

Easing factors: does the patient respond positively to rest or analgesics?

Severity, Irritability, Nature (SIN): How severe is the pain (0–5)? How irritable is the pain; does it settle quickly with rest? What is the nature of the pain – myogenic, arthrogenic, neurogenic, inflammatory or something else?

Problem list

1 Left elbow joint pain.
2 Reduced left thoracic limb elbow ROM.
3 Muscle imbalance of the affected limb.
4 Reduced left thoracic limb weight-bearing and function.
5 Reduced muscle bulk/strength.
6 Impaired gait pattern.
7 Reduced stamina and fitness.

Goals

1 Reduce left elbow joint pain (2–6 weeks).
2 Improve left thoracic limb elbow ROM (6 weeks).
3 Improve muscle length and strength (6 weeks).
4 Improve weight-bearing and function of left thoracic limb (6 weeks).
5 Improve muscle bulk/strength (6 weeks).
6 Gait re-education (6–12 weeks).
7 Improve stamina and fitness (6–12 weeks).

Treatment

- Laser treatment of elbow joint to reduce pain and inflammation and control scar tissue.
- PROM exercises within comfortable range for the patient, three sets of 10 repetitions.
- Passive stretches of tight biceps and pectorals into resistance and hold for 15 seconds, repeat three times.
- Active exercises to encourage weight transfer onto the affected limb (weaving cones), and also to promote adduction and abduction of the limb.
- Cavaletti poles to encourage flexion and extension of the affected joint.
- Weight-bearing exercises over a physio *peanut ball*. By passively moving the peanut ball forwards and backwards the patient will place and take weight

through the affected limb. Passive side-to-side movement will encourage the patient to place and take weight through the limb laterally and medially. This exercise will also challenge and therefore improve balance and core stability.

- A UWT can be used to encourage weight-bearing and function of the affected limb; because of the buoyancy effect of the water less concussive forces will pass through the joints, plus the warmth of the water will mean the patient will find this a comfortable environment to exercise in.

A combination of active exercises, including the UWT, can be used to strengthen the muscles around the joint and improve bulk and therefore improve stability of the joint. The UWT is also useful to re-educate gait; the water level can be adjusted to encourage strengthening, and exercising in a water treadmill has also been shown to improve the ROM of joints. The speed of the belt can be increased to encourage the patient to take longer strides. The duration of time the patient exercises in the UWT can be increased to improve fitness and stamina; this can be further enhanced by using water jets to add in resistance.

Owner education will focus on gradually increasing the patient's level of activity in a controlled manner, so lead exercise only should be advised initially. At 6 weeks postoperatively a callus will begin to form and the limb should be stable enough to allow weight-bearing through the limb. However, the repaired fracture site will not be consolidated until 12 weeks, and remodelling of the fracture will continue for up to 12 months. Uncontrolled exercise and jumping should be strongly discouraged; until remodelling is complete exercises can be increased after a satisfactory 12-week check, and with the permission of the veterinary surgeon.

Evaluation

Aim to evaluate treatment and the patient's progress at regular intervals. If he is not progressing as expected question if you need to change your treatment approach or should he be reassessed by the veterinary surgeon if his condition is not improving as expected.

Progression

Assuming the patient is improving and achieving the goals drawn up from the problem list it is important to progress his rehabilitation programme to prevent him plateauing. Remember, the overall aim of the rehabilitation programme is to return the patient to his highest level of function without ongoing disability. Progression may be to increase the speed of the exercises, add in more weaving cones to encourage weight transfer onto the affected limb, or increase the height of the cavaletti poles to increase elbow flexion ROM. Note that all exercises should be graded and gradually increased as over-exercise may cause exacerbation of symptoms.

Outcome measures

1. Outcome measures should be taken at the initial assessment to record baseline, and re-measured to assess the patient's progress at week 6, when changes in muscle mass can be expected, and repeated again at discharge, which in many cases would be around week 12.
2. Use a pain measure scale to evaluate the pain score.
3. Measure PROM of the affected elbow using a goniometer (flexion and extension), and compare with the contralateral limb.
4. Measure weight-bearing through limbs; it is worth measuring all four limbs. Knowing where the patient is shifting his weight from the affected limb is useful in identifying possible secondary complications occurring in the overloaded limb.
5. Measure muscle bulk of the affected limb with a tape measure, and compare with the contralateral limb. Aim to take the measure from the belly of the biceps/triceps muscle for consistency; moreover, as the patient builds muscle mass this will show around the muscle belly.
6. Video gait pattern at initial assessment, and use this to compare the gait pattern over time as the patient progresses.
7. Measuring heart and respiratory rate before and after exercise will give an indication of the patient's level of fitness.

CASE STUDY: PHYSIOTHERAPY REHABILITATION PROGRAMME FOR A FRACTURED RADIUS AND ULNA, LEFT THORACIC LIMB (OPEN, COMMINUTED)

Introduction

Otis is a 6-year-old, male, neutered lurcher.

Clinical history

Otis presented as an emergency; he had sustained an open fracture of his left thoracic limb after catching his foot in a hole whilst running. On presentation he was quiet but alert and was able to stand on his other three limbs.

Investigations

Preanaesthetic blood work did not reveal any significant abnormalities.

Radiographs of the affected limb revealed a comminuted proximal diaphyseal radial fracture of the ulna and radius. Examination under general anaesthetic confirmed the open nature of the fractures. There was a large U-shaped wound on the flexor surface of the left elbow region with avulsion of the skin from the underlying subcutaneous tissue (Figure 1.10).

Diagnosis

Fracture of the left thoracic limb – radius and ulna (open, comminuted).

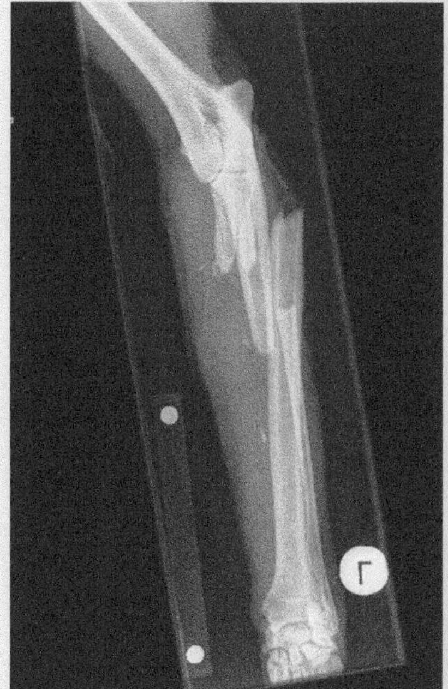

Figure 1.10 A left cranio-caudal fractured radius and ulna.

Surgery

A 1.6-mm Steinmann pin was placed in retrograde fashion to restore ulnar alignment. A modified type 1B external skeletal fixator was applied with one full pin through the olecranon, one half pin laterally in the proximal ulna, and four half pins in the mid to distal diaphysis and metaphysis. It was not possible to apply fixation to the proximal radius due to the presence of multiple fissure lines. Prior to closure a cancellous bone graft was harvested from the ipsilateral proximal humerus and applied to the radial fracture site. Antebrachial muscle and subcutaneous tissue was closed with 3/0 PDS® (polydioxanone) Suture (Ethicon) in simple interrupted pattern (Figure 1.11).

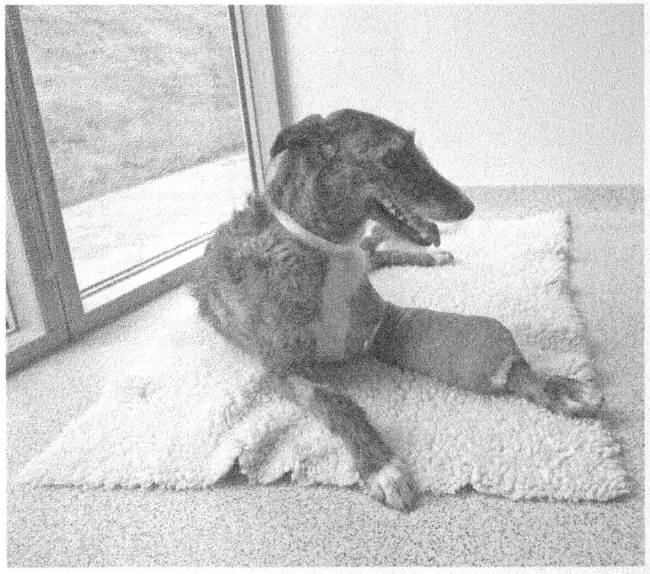

Figure 1.11 Post-fracture repair. The image shows the patient following surgery with a dressing on the left thoracic limb.

Reassessment

Otis presented for reassessment 6 weeks after antebrachial fracture repair. He was found to be only weight-bearing on the affected limb perhaps 10% of the time and showed generalised muscle atrophy of the brachium. The carpus and elbow had reduced ROM.

Investigations

Radiographs taken under sedation revealed maintenance of apposition and alignment and progression of fracture healing (Figure 1.12). Palpation revealed no instability at the radial fracture site.

Comment

Otis's fractures had healed sufficiently for the fixator to be removed. It was hoped that the use of his affected limb would gradually improve and he was referred for physiotherapy to encourage this. Ongoing remodelling at the

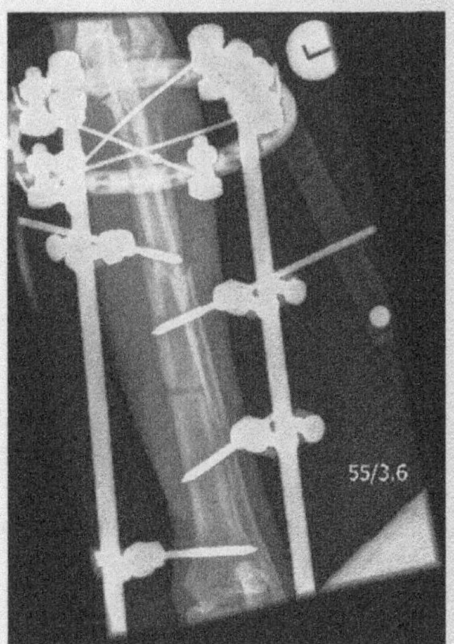

Figure 1.12 A left cranio-caudal radius and ulna repair.

fracture site was expected so his exercise at home was restricted to on-lead activity for the next 4–5 weeks.

History

On presentation Otis was partial weight-bearing through the left thoracic limb; however, he remained considerably lame. He had a short left forelimb stride with reduced left elbow and carpal flexion during gait. There was muscle atrophy of the left triceps and deltoid muscles. He had relatively good ROM of the left elbow with almost full extension and 140° of flexion with some discomfort at end of range. Left carpal flexion was reduced by 20° most likely as a result of soft tissue shortening and scar tissue. In addition Otis had soft tissue tension in the musculature of the right thoracic limb as a result of over using that limb to compensate for the left thoracic limb.

Physiotherapy assessment

Subjective

The owner reported that Otis is doing well with short lead walks.

Objective

- *Gait* – lame left thoracic limb 2/5 (scale 0–5), pain limits function.
- *Joint ROM* – hyperextension of left carpus 220°, flexion reduced 20°.
- *Muscle mass* – atrophy of left triceps, and deltoid 3 cm difference between right and left thoracic limb, mild muscle tension in right biceps, triceps and deltoid.

Problem list

1. Pain in the affected left limb.
2. Reduced ROM in the left carpus.
3. Muscle imbalance in the left thoracic limb.
4. Reduced function in the affected left limb with compensatory muscle tension in contralateral right limb.
5. Reduced strength in the left thoracic limb.
6. Altered gait pattern.
7. Reduced fitness.

Goals

1 Reduce pain (2 weeks).
2 Improve ROM (2–6 weeks).
3 Improve muscle imbalance (6 weeks).
4 Improve function and reduce compensatory muscle tension (6 weeks).
5 Improve strength (6–12 weeks).
6 Gait re-education (6–12 weeks).
7 Improve fitness/stamina (6–12 weeks).

Treatment

- Laser treatment of the fracture site and carpus to reduce pain and inflammation.
- Left carpal soft tissue release (STR), to regain normal ROM of the carpal joint.
- Left carpal mobilisations, grade II-III, 3 × 10 to reduce pain and improve ROM of the carpal joint.
- Biceps, internal rotators, and carpal stretches on the left thoracic limb into resistance and hold for 20 seconds, repeat three times (*N.B. Note the longer hold time for shortened soft tissues*).
- Right thoracic limb STR, to reduce muscle tension.
- Weaving cones 6 × 6, to improve weight transfer and abduction and adduction of the affected limb.
- Cavaletti poles 6 × 6 at 15 m height – reduced left carpal flexion, compensation from shoulder noted.
- Wobble board with limb lifting, increased extension left carpus noted, when additional weight passing through the limb.
- Hydrotherapy using an underwater treadmill 4 × 4 minutes at 6 kmp with resistance, water to the level of the elbows, good movement of left thoracic limb in the water observed.

Analysis (conclusion)

Reduced ROM, strength and function, post radius and ulna fracture repair; pain limits function. Consider using a carpal splint to improve ROM, function and strength of the affected limb.

Evaluate treatment

- Pain score at 6 and 12 weeks and compare with baseline measures.
- Measure passive joint ROM (compare with right thoracic limb) at 6 and 12 weeks.
- Measure muscle bulk (compare with right thoracic limb) at 6 and 12 weeks.
- Measure percent weight-bearing through limbs (compare with baseline measures, taken at initial assessment, measure at week 6 and 12).
- Gait assessment and score lameness, video gait at baseline, compare at 6 and 12 weeks to evaluate effectiveness of physiotherapy programme (Video 1.3).

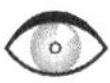

Progress treatment

- Increase length of walks and add in inclines, to improve stamina and strength.
- Introduce stairs, as a functional activity.
- Increase the speed and duration of time exercising in the hydrotherapy sessions.

VIDEO 1.3

Gait/lameness scoring. When the patient walks towards the camera a mild lameness and head bob can be seen in the affected left thoracic limb, which is also hyperextended. At trot this is more obvious and the patient's head bob is more obvious. Gait lameness score grade 2/5.

Tendon injuries

Tendon injuries result from a partial or complete rupture of the muscle-tendon junction. These injuries involve over-stretching of the muscle-tendon fibres and are often traumatic in origin; they are seen most frequently in sporting breeds such as racing greyhounds.

Conservative treatment can be effective for mild tendon injuries, using the PRICE regime (Figure 1.13).

Surgical tendon injuries

Acute lacerations and avulsion tendon injuries usually require surgical intervention. The goal is to try to gain good apposition of the two ends of tendon to avoid excessive scar tissue, which can lead to

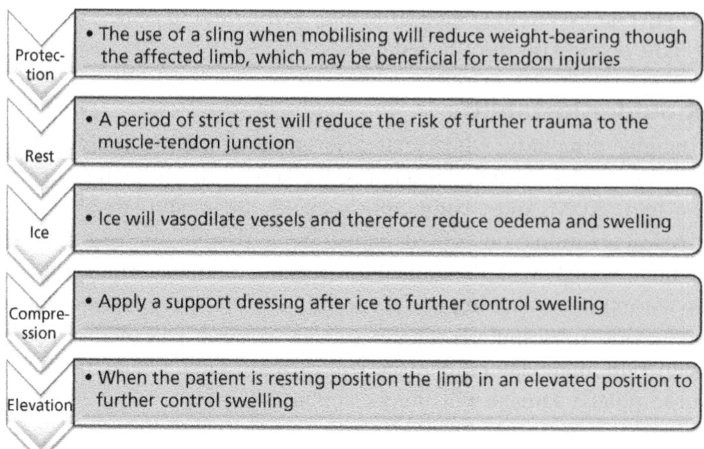

Figure 1.13 The PRICE regime for conservative treatment of musculoskeletal injuries.

adhesions and shortening of the tendon. Tendon and ligaments also tend to have a poor blood supply, meaning they can take a long time to heal and regain tensile strength.

Postoperatively a cast is usually applied to offer protection to the tendon repair. The cast may be applied to prevent loading of the affected limb and to keep the tendon repair in a shortened state. This cast would usually be left in place for 6 weeks and the usual cast care criteria would apply. If there is a lot of associated soft tissue swelling postoperatively the original cast may be reapplied within the first week, as the swelling subsides the cast will become lose and may cause skin irritation and tissue ulceration.

When the cast is removed and the veterinary surgeon is happy with the tendon repair gentle PROM exercises and stretches may begin. When the tendon is cast in a shortened position this will also affect the associated muscles, which will become short and tight.

It may take weeks of graded stretching of the limb to achieve normal weight-bearing on the affected limb.

Shoulder instability

Shoulder instability, which may also be described as shoulder subluxation or glenohumeral instability, is characterised by an increase in the joint ROM, most commonly seen in the medio-lateral plane. Physical examination will demonstrate a passive increase of the abduction angle with the animal in lateral recumbency. This is caused by tearing or weakening of the medial or lateral glenohumeral ligaments and subscapularis tendon (medial damage will increase limb abduction angle, lateral damage will increase limb adduction angle, subscapularis damage will affect scapular stability).

Conservative treatment

- 6–12 weeks restricted exercise.
- Analgesia.
- Physiotherapy aims to strengthen the muscles around the shoulder joint to reduce instability and reduce the risk of associated secondary osteoarthritis.

Physiotherapy plan

Laser therapy is applied using a continuous movement pattern directly over the affected area. In the early stages the aim is to reduce pain and inflammation. In the later stages the aim is to reduce adhesions and shortening of tissues associated with excessive scar tissue.

Weaving cones can encourage limb abduction and adduction. Start with the cones spread far apart then as the patient progresses bring the cones closer together.

Walking in figures-of-eight and circles will increase abduction and adduction. Again, start with wide circles and figures, and as the patient progresses lead in smaller circles and figures-of-eight.

Place a wobble cushion under the affected limb; this unstable surface will challenge the subscapularis muscle and work to stabilise the scapula. Challenge the patient further by incorporating limb lifting of the contralateral thoracic limb, then the contralateral pelvic limb. Remember to support the patient under the abdomen and trunk as necessary. As the patient progresses further a wobble board may be used, this can be used to target and challenge abduction and adduction of the affected limb, by rocking the board medially and laterally; as the patient resists this motion he will strengthen his abductors and adductors. Rocking the board forwards and backwards with the animal facing forwards will load the limbs in a cranio-caudal plane. The wobble board also improves core stability and challenges balance. It is most effective if introduced slowly so the patient can become accustomed to the equipment; start with short sessions. As the patient progresses limb lifting can be incorporated to challenge the patient further. Remember to support the patient under the abdomen and trunk as necessary. If the patient feels secure he is more likely to accept the equipment and exercise.

Hydrotherapy using a UWT can be used in the acute stage to encourage weight-bearing through the affected limb. The buoyancy effect of the water can be used to reduce the load passing through the limb. At this stage the level of the water should be at approximately mid-trunk. The speed of the treadmill belt should be less than the patient's normal gait speed to encourage use of the affected limb.

As the patient progresses the water can be used to provide resistance and the level of the water should be set to mid humerus as; the most resistance is at the water surface. The speed of the treadmill belt can be gradually increased over a period of weeks to increase stamina, and resistance from water jets may be used to further increase strength.

In the early stages (first 6 weeks) stretches of the structures around the shoulder joint should be avoided. The ligaments supporting this joint are already overstretched and weak. Gentle stretching may commence after 6 weeks if there is reduced passive ROM of the shoulder joint associated with soft tissue shortening. Note that joint passive ROM may also be reduced if the patient has osteoarthritis in the affected joint.

Surgical intervention aims to reconstruct the ligaments supporting the shoulder joint. The challenges of reconstructing the ligaments of the shoulder joint are similar to those in other limb ligament reconstructions. Tendons take a long time to heal; weight-bearing should be avoided for 6 weeks postoperatively to avoid loading the fragile ligament repair.

Active physiotherapy would usually commence following a satisfactory 6-week postoperative check from the veterinary surgeon. The physiotherapy plan following surgical reconstruction of the ligaments would aim to strengthen muscles around the shoulder joint, improve weight-bearing and function of the affected limb. Challenge balance, and address any secondary compensatory issues the patient may have adopted from the original injury.

Biceps tenosynovitis

Biceps tenosynovitis results from inflammation of the biceps brachii tendon, which may be the result of direct or indirect trauma to the bicipital tendon. Often the cause may be related to repetitive use or over-use and is therefore often seen in agility and sporting breeds. The biceps tendon is a stabiliser of the shoulder joint, and biceps tenosynovitis may occur in conjunction with generalised shoulder instability.

Physical examination

Gait: the animal will usually present lame on the affected limb, with abduction of the limb to reduce weight-bearing; reduced ROM at the shoulder joint to reduce pain and inflammation around the tendon and sheath may be observed.

Palpation: direct palpation over the tendon using the back of the hand may indicate heat – a sign of inflammation; this should be compared with the non-affected limb. The tendon itself may also feel thickened when compared to the non-affected limb.

ROM: may be reduced as a result of adhesions and excessive fibrous tissue forming around the tendon and its sheath.

Pain: end-of-range flexion of the shoulder joint will produce pain as the tendon will be fully stretched. Osteophytes may form within the intertubercular groove causing further irritation and inflammation of the tendon.

Radiography: changes may be unremarkable in the acute stage as osteophytes do not form until the later more chronic stage.

Arthroscopy: will demonstrate tendon disease including thickening and inflammation.

Conservative treatment

- Prednisolone injection into the bicipital tendon sheath (oral prednisolone does not appear to be affective).
- Rest followed by graded, controlled exercise.

Surgical treatment

Bicipital tendon tenotomy or tenodesis generally is associated with good outcomes. The recovery period following surgical treatment is 2–9 months to regain optimal function. Physiotherapy can commence following a satisfactory 6-week postoperative check from the veterinary surgeon.

Physiotherapy

- Laser therapy over the biceps tendon to reduce any inflammation.
- PROM exercises to maintain ROM in the affected limb.
- Stretches to maintain muscle length; do not take the biceps stretch to end of range as this will be painful for the patient.
- Frictions directly over the biceps tendon in a medio-lateral direction 3 × 30 seconds; in the acute phase avoid being too vigorous with friction treatment as this will be uncomfortable for the

patient. Frictions aim to break down adhesions around the tendon and sheath and should be followed with careful stretching of the biceps muscle and tendon.

Active exercises

- Weaving cones to encourage weigh transfer on the affected limb.
- Cavaletti poles to improve ROM and proprioception of the affected limb.
- Stairs are a functional exercise; note that descending stairs may be painful in the early stages as the patient will be fully loading the affected limb so this may be an exercise to avoid in the early stages to prevent exacerbation of the biceps tendon.
- Wobble cushions placed under the affected limb will improve strength around the stabilising muscles of the shoulder. This can be progressed by lifting the contralateral thoracic limb or the contralateral pelvic limb as the patient progresses; remember to support the patient under the abdomen and trunk as necessary.
- Wobble board. As the patient progresses further the wobble board can be used to improve strength and stability of the muscles around the affected shoulder joint as the patient resists the movement of the board.
- Hydrotherapy using an underwater treadmill to provide buoyancy will encourage the patient to use the limb functionally and improve ROM of the affected limb. As the animal progresses the level of the water can be adjusted to strengthen the muscles around the shoulder joint and the water level should be set to mid-humerus. The speed of the treadmill belt can be increased to increase stride length, and the duration of sessions can be increased to improve stamina. Finally, resistance from the water jets can be added to improve strengthening.

Outcome measures

Measure baseline ROM of the affected limb using a goniometer; compare against the unaffected limb. Re-measure at 6 and 12 weeks to evaluate progress.

Measure baseline muscle mass, using a tape measure around the muscle belly of the biceps and triceps muscle; compare this against the unaffected limb. Re-measure at 6 and 12 weeks to evaluate progress.

Video gait pattern and score lameness at assessment and record these baseline measures, then re-measure at 6 and 12 weeks to evaluate progress.

Assess weight bearing through the limb

- *Subjective* – how easy is it to pick up the affected limb?
- *Objective* – using a pressure-sensitive analysis mat or bathroom weighing scales will also give an idea of where the patient is shifting his weight, indicating that he is placing additional stress on these limbs, and may be at risk of developing secondary compensatory complications. Measure baseline at assessment; re-measure at 6 and 12 weeks to evaluate progress.

Pain management

Multimodal approach

An understanding of the patient's pathology is essential when considering a pain management approach. Excellent handling skills when moving and assisting patients to mobilise will minimise pain and lead to an earlier return to function with reduced secondary complications such as muscle imbalances or the development of abnormal postures.

Gate control theory

The gate control theory (Figure 1.14) was first introduced by Melzack and Wall (1965). Three types of fibres are associated with the gate control theory:

- A-delta fibres.
- C fibres.
- A-beta fibres.

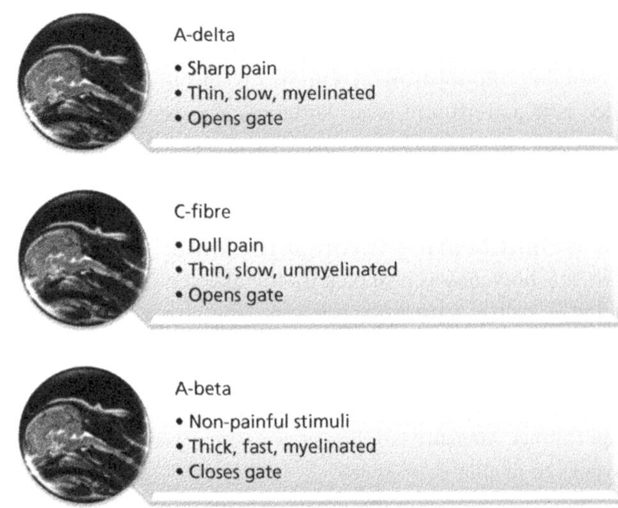

Figure 1.14 Gate control theory.

A-delta fibres transmit sharp, prickly pain signals; the fibres are thin and myelinated, and transmission is slow. C fibres transmit a dull, aching pain signal; the fibres are thin and unmyelinated, and transmission is slow. When stimulated A-delta and C fibres open the pain control 'gate' and pain is perceived in the brain.

A-beta fibres when stimulated can act on inhibitory neurons to block transmission of painful stimuli via the A-delta and C fibres to the brain. A-beta fibres are large, thick and myelinated, and they transmit fast signals. When A-beta fibres are stimulated the gate is closed and pain is not perceived in the brain.

It is thought that TENS machines control or modulate pain perception by stimulating the A-beta fibres, and inhibiting input from the A-delta and C fibres.

Also many naturally occurring substances can inhibit pain perception:

- Endogenous opioids (encephalins, endorphins).
- Adenosine.
- Norepinephrine.
- Dopamine.

Severity

Consideration should be given to the severity of pain. Many human pain scales are available such as the visual analog scale (VAS); this is a pain measure scale ranging from 0 to 10, where 0 would be the patient's perception of no pain whatsoever, and 10 would correspond to the worst pain imaginable by the patient. The VAS has been shown to have excellent validity and reliability in humans. However, the VAS could not be applied to animal patients, as they are unable to give subjective feedback. An alternative is the Glasgow composite measure pain scale – short form (GCMPS-SF).

The GCMPS-SF has been shown to be a valid measure of pain in animals and has intra-rater (observer) reliability. Valid and reliable measures of the severity of the patient's pain will guide the veterinary surgeon when administering analgesics. The GCMPS-SF should be used in conjunction with the expected duration of analgesics administered. For example, if the analgesic has a 4-hour duration of effectiveness, the GCMPS-SF should be completed at the end of the 4 hours. The score of the GCMPS-SF will guide the veterinary surgeon in his or her choice of analgesics. If the pain appears under control the same analgesic regime may be continued in the early postoperative stage, or a decision may be made to taper the dose of analgesia, or to switch from a pure opioid to a partial opioid.

A simple pain score scale (0–4) can be useful for grading pain during the physical examination when manipulating the affected joint (Table 1.4).

Table 1.4 Pain score scale 0–4.

Score	Description
0	No signs of pain during manipulation of the affected joint
1	Signs of mild pain during palpation of joint
2	Signs of moderate pain during palpation
3	Signs of severe pain during palpation
4	Dog will not allow examiner to palpate joint

Irritability

The irritability of pain should also be considered. The irritability of pain is related to the duration of pain. For example, the pain experienced by the patient may be severe, but relatively short lived; if this is the case a potent analgesic may be selected, but only a short duration of analgesia is required. This is worth considering if the animal has undesirable side effects from opioid analgesics. Pain would be considered as irritable if once triggered the level of pain takes several hours to settle. In this case an analgesic with a long duration of action would be selected.

Nature

The nature of pain is another consideration. *Myogenic* or *muscular pain* is described in humans as a dull, aching pain. It tends to have a VAS of around 5/10 and is often related to fatigue or overuse. Myogenic pain can last for several hours but it responds well to rest and heat therapy if spasm is a feature of the pain.

Inflammatory pain may be associated with stiffness. This may be seen early in the morning when the animal rises. Gentle movement and controlled exercise can reduce the pain. Inflammatory pain is also associated with surgery; the veterinary surgeon may use a short course of NSAIDs in conjunction with opioids in these cases.

Neurogenic pain can be associated with sharp, shooting pains, and altered sensation and loss of function in humans. The severity and irritability of neurogenic pain can vary. Accurate pain scoring using a valid and reliable measuring tool will guide the veterinary surgeon in choosing an appropriate analgesic regime for each individual patient.

Many other types of pain are recognised in humans, and many types of analgesics are available to relieve pain. A multimodal approach is most beneficial as often myogenic, inflammatory and neurogenic pain can co-exist within a single patient. Severity and irritability must be considered when using a pain measuring tool such as the GCMPS-SF as these are dynamic variables.

Analgesics

The analgesic regime will be devised and regularly reviewed by the veterinary surgeon. The veterinary nurse should be confident in using pain measuring tools and reporting any changes in the patient's pain level to the veterinary surgeon.

Physiotherapy musculoskeletal assessment

Ensure familiarity with the surgical procedure or condition of the patient; liaise with the veterinary surgeon if in any doubt.

Gait: assess the patient's weight-bearing status through the affected limb(s). Is he NWB, PWB or FWB? Is this what you would expect to find? For example, NWB status would be expected in the early rehabilitation phase, PWB in the mid-phase, and FWB in the late phase.

Palpate the surgical site for signs of inflammation (redness, swelling, pain, heat)/infection, and loss of function. Again inflammation is to be expected in the early phase, but not in the mid and late phases. Infection should not be present at any stage and should be reported to the veterinary surgeon immediately.

Joint ROM: This may be reduced in the early phase and ROM may be limited by inflammation and pain. In the mid-phase joint ROM should improve as inflammation and pain subside. In the late phase joint ROM should be normal for that patient, providing he has received adequate rehabilitation. *N.B. If osteoarthritis is present or developing secondary to surgical intervention ROM will be reduced at end of range, and a bony end feel will be noted; the patient will feel discomfort at this point.*

Muscle length: Muscles can become imbalanced if the patient has prolonged lameness and reduced function in the affected limb. Muscles often work in pairs, so if the triceps in the thoracic limb becomes weak, because the patient is NWB on this limb, the opposing biceps muscle, which will be contracted to hold the limb in flexion, will become short and tight. During the early phase of rehabilitation NWB status is desirable; however, with sling support PWB status is desirable in the mid-rehabilitation phase to minimise muscle imbalance associated with long-term misuse of a limb. In the late phase of rehabilitation normal muscle length without imbalances should be achieved.

Muscle bulk/strength: Muscle bulk should be measured with a tape measure around the circumference of the limb at the level of the muscle belly, as this is where changes in muscle mass will be most apparent. Measure three times and use the average measure; compare the measure against the non-affected contralateral limb where possible. Record these measures as *baseline.* This outcome measure should be repeated at 6 and 12 weeks to evaluate progress.

Muscle tone: may be described as:

Normal tone is the resistance expected when the limb(s) are passively flexed and extended.

Hypertonic tone is when increased resistance is observed during passive limb flexion and extension exercises.

Hypotonic tone is when decreased resistance is observed during passive limb flexion and extension exercises.

Posture: This is the observation of the patient's alignment and body symmetry. If the patient is lame his alignment and symmetry will change; if this change in alignment is not addressed secondary complications or compensatory postures may develop.

Secondary complications/compensatory postures: Secondary complications include muscle imbalances, which may be associated with altered function and weight-bearing through the limbs. Compensatory postures can develop if a patient has a prolonged period of lameness leading to poor posture and alignment with associated *trigger points* in the compensating overused muscle groups. Secondary complications and compensatory postures can lead to chronic pain. Patients who develop compensatory postures may demonstrate:

Kyphosis – defined as an abnormal curve or flexion of the spine, usually in the thoracic spine. It may be caused by abnormal vertebrae or by a developmental abnormality. Animals who present with a lesion in the thoracic spine will often adopt a kyphotic posture; this may be an attempt to relieve pressure from an intervertebral disc protrusion or extrusion. This posture is also often observed in the patient following hemi-laminectomy and decompression of the spinal cord, the surgery itself is very invasive and a degree of swelling and inflammation around the surgical site is normal. Over time the swelling and inflammation will subside and the patient's spinal posture should become normal again.

Lordosis – refers to an inward curve usually in the lumbar spine.

Scoliosis – is an abnormal curvature of the spine to either the right or left side.

Subjective examination

The subjective examination focuses on information obtained from the owner, or on something you have read in the medical notes. It may be useful to record this information on a body chart.

- *Localisation of symptoms:* The aim is to identify the painful areas. For example, if the patient has hip dysplasia mark this on the chart as *pain a*; if this is a chronic condition the patient may well have referred pain in the lumbar spine as a result of secondary compensatory issues, so mark this on the chart as *pain b.* Generally 'pain a' will be more severe than 'pain b', so if 'pain a' can be controlled 'pain b' will tend to resolve also.

- *Intensity of pain:* Ask the owner how lame the patient is. The owner may inform you that the patient is stiff in the morning when he rises but then 'walks it off' as the day progresses. Is the patient guarding the affected area? Is he reluctant to be examined? Score for pain and lameness.
- *Intermittent or constant?* Is the pain intermittent and if so does it relate to exercise levels? Or does the patient appear to be in constant pain? Constant pain would indicate a high level of irritability and his analgesia may need to be reviewed by the veterinary surgeon. Ask about easing and aggravating factors i.e is rest or exercise a factor.
- *Abnormal sensation (numbness):* Does the animal respond to changes in temperature? Can he distinguish between hot and cold? Does he have a normal withdrawal reflex when you 'pinch' between his toes? Is it the same when compared to the contralateral limb?
- *Relationship of symptoms:* If the patient presents with lameness, is it the cause of the spinal pain, or is the lameness an effect of the spinal pain? If the lameness is the cause of spinal pain the limb pain is the primary pain, and the spinal pain is secondary, or sometimes classed as referred pain. However, if the spinal pain is causing the lameness the spinal pain is the primary pain and the limb pain is the secondary pain. As a general rule the primary pain will be more severe than secondary pain. Palpate the individual areas and pain score them separately to distinguish between primary and secondary (referred pain).
- *Check other relevant regions:* If the patient presents lame on the thoracic limb but no pain can be localised in the limb, check for cervical spine pain, which may be the primary cause of the lameness.

Behaviour of symptoms

- *Aggravating factors* –the lameness may be associated with long walks, or lying in one position for a long time, then the patient may be stiff to rise.
- *Easing factors* – symptoms may improve with rest, or if heat is applied to the affected area.

- *Severity* – this is closely linked with the intensity of symptoms; pain score for a baseline measure then re-measure at regular intervals to evaluate progress.
- *Irritability* – this is linked to the duration of the pain; i.e. if the patient rests or heat is applied to the affected area do the painful symptoms decrease? If the pain decreases quickly it is not very irritable; however. if the pain lasts for several hours or even days it would be classed as very irritable.

  Pain severity and irritability are often correlates; e.g. pain from a recent fracture fixation would be considered to be severe and irritable. However, over time both the severity and irritability of pain would normally decrease.
- *Daily activities/functional limitations* – how much exercise does the patient usually have? Does the patient have to climb stairs to go outside? Can he jump in and out of the car?
- *24-hour behaviour* – does the pain disturb the patient's sleep? Does he seem more painful first thing in the morning, or does the pain develop through the day? Inflammatory type pain disturbs sleep and is common early in the morning. However, as the patient begins to move around the pain and stiffness generally ease. Myogenic pain tends not to be severe, and is described as a dull aching pain in humans. It may be related to overuse, and will usually reduce with rest. Neurogenic pain is severe and it may or may not be irritable. It is worth noting that several different types of pain can co-exist in a single patient at the same time, so a multimodal approach to pain relief will be required.
- *Stage of the condition* – is it an acute or chronic injury? Is the condition improving, staying the same or getting worse? If the condition is improving continue with the same treatment. If the condition is static it may be that the patient has reached a plateau, so the treatment should be changed or progressed. If the patient is getting worse change the treatment; maybe go back a step if the rehabilitation programme is too advanced for him, or refer him back to his veterinary surgeon for a review.

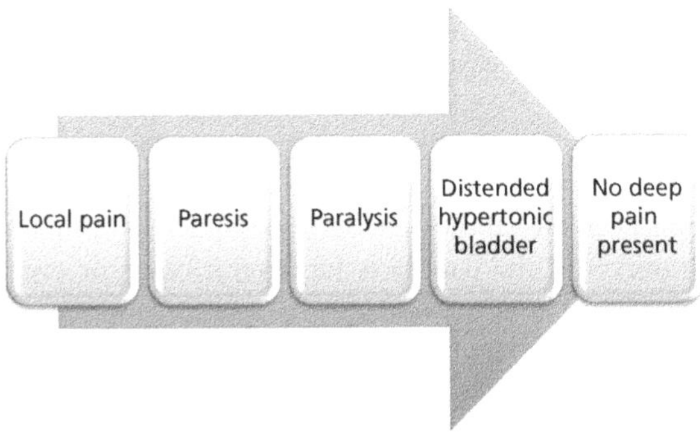

Figure 1.15 Progressive signs of spinal cord or cauda equina symptoms.

Special questions

Does the patient have spinal cord or cauda equina symptoms? If so urgent bladder management will be required, followed by an immediate referral to a neurologist (Figure 1.15).

History of present condition (HPC)

- *Mechanism of injury* – did the owner observe the injury, i.e. 'the dog jumped to catch the ball, twisted awkwardly, cried out in pain, and was immediately weak on the back leg.'
- *Change of each symptom since onset* – is the pain getting better, staying the same, or getting worse?
- *Recent X-rays or investigation* – review findings and discuss with colleagues as necessary.

Past medical history (PMH)

- Relevant medical history.
- Previous episodes of present complaint.
- Previous treatment and outcome.
- General health.

Drug history (DH)

- Current medication.
- Steroids.
- Note any allergies.

Social history (SH)

- Age and gender.
- Home situation (stairs, access to garden, other pets and children in the household).
- Exercise (normal level pre-injury or -illness).

Physical examination

Observation

- *Posture* – weight shifting off affected limb(s).
- *Function* – ability to climb stairs, or jump in and out of car.
- *Gait* – ability to walk, trot and run.
- *Structural abnormalities* – kyphosis, lordosis, scoliosis.
- *Muscle bulk and tone* – measure muscle circumference and compare with contralateral limb. Is the muscle tone high, normal or low?
- *Soft tissue* – assess for signs of pain/trigger points. Assess muscle length/imbalance.

Passive joint movements

- Passive joint ROM – measure in degrees using goniometer.
- Joint effusion measurement, using a tape measure and compare with contralateral limb.

Muscle tests

- *Muscle strength, control and stability* – can use limb lifting with support as necessary to test how much weight is passing through the affected limb, or by observation of functional activities, such as stairs, which challenge strength, control and stability.
- *Muscle length* – assess by passively stretching muscles; observe any 'tightness' or muscle contractures, which may be common in muscles that cross two joints such as biceps and quadriceps.

Neurological tests

If indicated test:

- Reflexes.
- Conscious proprioception.
- Withdrawal.
- Sensation.

Palpation

- Palpate the skin and superficial soft tissues – assess for heat (use back of hand, compare with contralateral limb) and oedema.
- Palpate muscles and tendons – assess for muscle tension or *trigger points*, assess tendons for signs of inflammation or abnormal tracking.
- Ligaments – assess stability and note any laxity.
- Joints – assess for pain and stiffness.
- Bones – note any abnormalities, i.e. limb valgus or varus.

Self-assessment questions

1 In cases of hip dysplasia, which passive movement of the coxofemoral (hip) joint is usually most restricted and painful?

a Flexion
b Extension
c Adduction
d External rotation

2 If an animal is 5/5 lame in the left pelvic limb for more than 2 weeks, what changes can be expected in the affected limb?

a Generalised muscle atrophy, tight hip flexors, and weak hamstrings.
b Generalised muscle atrophy, weak hip flexors, with strong hamstrings.
c An increase in muscle mass.
d No muscle changes.

3 Incomplete ossification of the humeral condyle (IOHC) is a condition mostly seen in:

a Labradors
b German shepherd dogs

c Toy poodles
d Springer spaniels

4 When considering the pain gate control theory, which of the following would lead to pain perception in the brain?
a Adenosine
b Norepinephrine
c C fibre stimulation
d Dopamine

5 Which of the following inhibits pain perception in the brain?
a A-delta fibres
b A-beta fibres
c C-fibres
d Projection cells

6 Which of the following is not considered to be a strengthening exercise?
a Underwater treadmill walking
b Swimming
c Stair climbing
d Passive range of motion exercises

7 When using electrotherapy, when must dark-green lens glasses be worn for eye protection?
a TENS machine
b Laser machine
c PEME therapy
d Therapeutic ultrasound machine

8 Which of the following is not a naturally occurring opioid?
a Methadone
b Encephalin
c Endorphin
d Dynorphin

9 Which exercise would most challenge a patient's balance?
a Walking around weaving cones.
b Weight-bearing through a limb placed on a wobble cushion.
c Stepping over cavaletti poles.
d The patient standing with all four limbs on a moving wobble board.

10 What is the sequence of cranial cruciate disease events?
  a Stifle instability, articular cartilage degeneration, capsular fibrosis, reduced ROM.
  b Articular cartilage degeneration, stifle instability, capsular fibrosis, reduced ROM.
  c Stifle instability, articular cartilage degeneration, reduced ROM, capsular fibrosis.
  d Stifle instability, capsular fibrosis, reduced stifle ROM, articular cartilage degeneration.

CHAPTER 2
Neurology

Introduction

Veterinary medicine is a progressive profession. Over the years more and more challenging neurological patients are being treated. It is equally important for veterinary nursing and physiotherapy to advance to support and rehabilitate these complex patients back to their highest level of function.

Undergoing spinal surgery is only part of the patient pathway. The patient will require nursing support to aid his recovery and physiotherapy to achieve optimum performance postoperatively. By adopting a patient-centred approach the veterinary team can work together to achieve the best outcome for the patient.

Key features of upper and lower motor neuron lesions

Upper motor neurons originate in the cerebral cortex, and terminate in the cranial nerve nuclei or spinal cord anterior horn. Signs and symptoms of upper motor neuron lesions are commonly seen in animals with head trauma resulting in brain injury.

Practical Physiotherapy for Veterinary Nurses, First Edition. Donna Carver.

Lower motor neurons originate in cranial nerve nuclei or in the spinal cord anterior horn, and terminate in skeletal muscle motor units. Signs and symptoms of lower motor neuron lesions are commonly seen with traumatic injuries such as brachial plexus evulsions.

Decreased muscle tone may be described as low tone, or hypotonicity. When the operator passively moves the affected limb(s) through range of motion (ROM) very little resistance to the movement will be appreciated.

Muscle tone may be increased, and described as high tone, or hypertonicity. When the affected limb(s) is passively moved through range of motion the operator will appreciate increased resistance to movements.

Clonus is an abnormal reflex seen in the affected animal in response to sudden passive dorsiflexion of the tarsus by the operator.

Tendon reflexes such as the patella reflex maybe increased, decreased or absent (Table 2.1).

Table 2.1 Features of upper and lower motor neuron lesions.

Feature	Upper motor neuron	Lower motor neuron
Muscle tone	Increased	Decreased
Clonus	Increased	Absent
Tendon reflexes	Increased	Decreased or absent
Distribution	Thoracic limb flexion increased, extension decreased Pelvic limb flexors decreased	Weakness of the muscle groups innervated by the affected spinal segment
Location	Brain, C1-5 and T3-L3 lesions	C6-T2, L4-S3 and neuromuscular lesions

Surgical presenting conditions

Intervertebral disc disease (IVDD)

IVDD Hansen type I

Hansen type I intervertebral disc disease (IVDD) tends to occur most frequently in chondrodystrophoid (dachshund, Lhasa apso) type breeds aged between 2 and 7 years with a peak incidence at 4–5 years old. The disc becomes cartilaginous, and its nucleus takes on a granular consistency resulting in a progressive loss of hydroelastic shock-absorbing qualities. The degenerative nucleus often undergoes calcification, further compromising its function. Traumatic events such as jumping and twisting may hasten the clinical signs of IVDD; however, once degeneration has progressed to a certain point, even normal activity can result in acute mechanical failure. This failure often results in complete rupture of the dorsal annulus and an explosive upward extrusion of a large volume of nuclear material into the vertebral canal (Slatter, 2003).

IVDD Hansen type II

Hansen type II intervertebral disc disease (IVDD) tends to occur in non-chondrodystrophoid breeds (Labrador retrievers, German shepherd dogs) later in life between 8 and 10 years of age, and generally causes less severe signs. The nucleus of the disc remains more gel-like and mineralisation is rare. Partial rupture of the annulus bands and bulging of the dorsal annulus results in a disc protrusion (Slatter, 2003) (Figure 2.1).

Medical management for IVDD

Medical management may be considered for cases that present with mild to moderate spinal pain and paraparesis, and also if the owner has financial restraints. Medical management consists of:

- Rest.
- Pain relief.

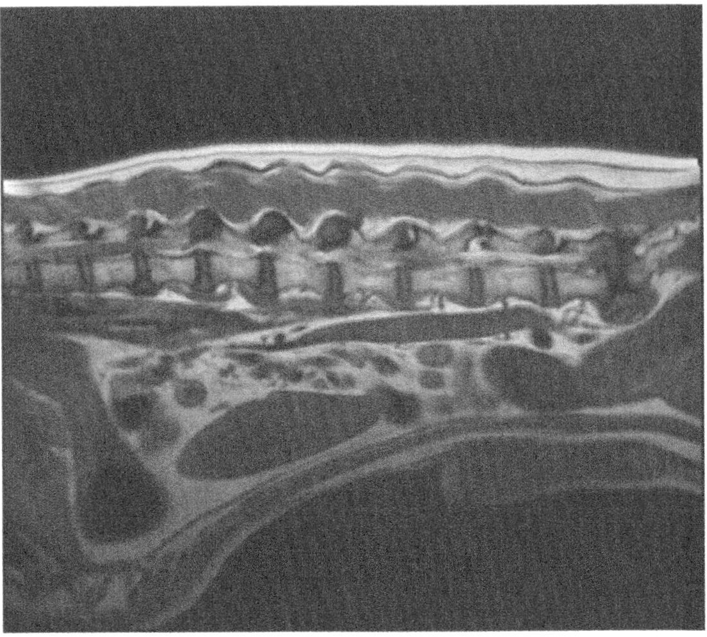

Figure 2.1 Chronic intervertebral disc disease at L1-2 with widespread cord compression.

- Gentle physiotherapy to maintain joint ROM, and muscle length.
- Heat packs to reduce muscle spasm (10–20 minutes, 3–4 times daily; use caution if the patient has altered temperature sensation).
- Standing and gait practice with support for toileting purposes only in the early stages.
- Progress the physiotherapy regime over weeks 4–6 if the pain is controlled; aim to strengthen pelvic limbs, and improve balance.

This type of management may be suited to Hansen type II disc protrusions, which tend to have a progressively chronic presentation.

Hansen type I disc extrusions tend to require surgical intervention based on acute presentation and severity of symptoms.

Surgical management for IVDD

Surgical management may be indicated if the patient is not responsive to medical management, or if the clinical signs progress to non-ambulatory paraparesis or paraplegia. Decompressive surgery for IVDD includes hemilaminectomy, dorsal laminectomy, or ventral slot for lesions in the cervical spine region.

Physiotherapy and rehabilitation plan for surgical patients (Hansen type I or II intervertebral disc disease)

Day 0

Day 0 is the day of surgery. Laser therapy, if available, may commence as the patient is recovering from surgery. Select the acute incision setting. NB do not use the laser over the thyroid area for ventral slot surgery, as lasering over the thyroid gland is contra-indicated.

The aim of laser therapy in this case is to promote healing of the incision site post-surgery. *Eye protection must be worn by the operator, and anyone else in close proximity to the laser beam.* Laser therapy of the surgical area should be repeated daily.

Day 1

Day 1 postoperative is considered a rest day. The patient is likely to be on opioid-based medication and non-steroidal anti-inflammatory drugs (NSAIDs). Nursing considerations are important and a waterproof mattress with absorbent bedding, such as vetbed® (Petlife International Ltd, Bury St Edmunds, Suffolk, UK) or a similar type, should be used to ensure the patient is comfortable and dry. The patient should be turned every 4 hours; if tolerated the patient may prefer to be in sternal recumbency, then just turn the hips. Ensure the patient is adequately supported when turning and avoid any rotation of the spinal column. Two people will be required to turn large dogs.

Aim to maintain good spinal alignment when turning a spinal patient and avoid twisting or rotating the spine during the manoeuvre.

If the surgical site is in the cervical spine region ensure the patient's head is supported when turning. If the patient is in the sternal position a small pad should be available for him to rest his head on to maintain a neural spinal position; do not elevate the head into extension.

The bladder should be palpated every 4 hours, and size and tension of the bladder noted. If the bladder is becoming large and tense, manual expression of the bladder may be necessary. If the veterinary surgeon is concerned about bladder function preoperatively he or she may place an indwelling urinary catheter at the end of surgery. This should be cleaned twice daily with a chlorhexidine solution, and the volume of urine should be measured every 4 hours to ensure urine production remains in the range 1–2 mL/kg/hour. Nursing of the patient will also include optimal nutrition for the recovering patient.

Laser therapy – repeat as for day 0; repeat daily until suture or staple removal.

If therapeutic laser is not available the veterinary surgeon may request:

Ice packing of the site every 4–6 hours; the aim is to reduce postoperative inflammation. An ice pack wrapped in a damp towel can be gently applied to the area for 10 minutes if tolerated by the patient. Also check with the veterinary surgeon beforehand as he or she may not wish for the surgical site to be interfered with. Ice packing is usually applied to the area every 4–6 hours for the first 72 hours post-surgery.

Positioning – if the patient is in lateral recumbency ensure a pad is placed between the thoracic limbs, and a second pad between the pelvic limbs to ensure the limbs remain in a neutral position and to prevent muscle imbalance. The internal rotator muscle groups tend to become short and tight and the external rotator muscle groups

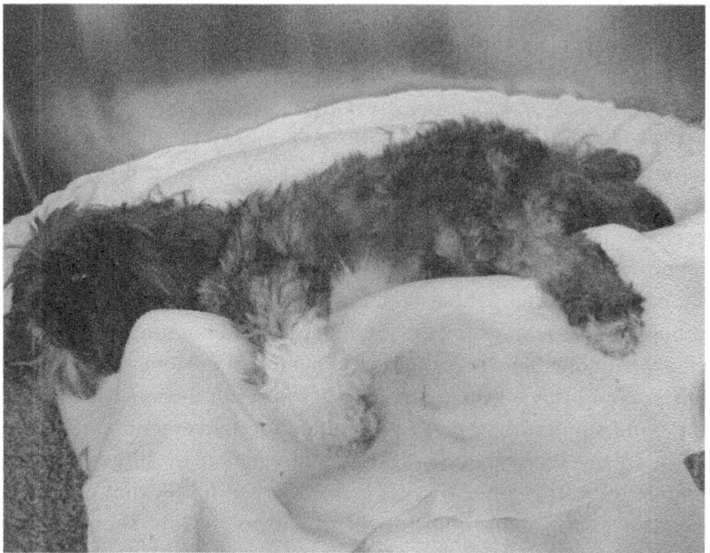

Figure 2.2 A tetraparetic patient positioned on his right side with his left limbs supported to prevent muscle imbalance (he is weaker on his left side).

tend to become long and weak, in non-ambulatory patients. Ensuring correct muscle length by supporting the patient with positioning aids aims to minimise this (Figure 2.2).

If the animal is in sternal recumbency, only his pelvic limbs will require turning and supporting in neutral with a pelvic wedge.

Standing – supported standing may be performed once on day 1. This is usually with the veterinary surgeon present as he or she will assess the patient's neurological status post-surgery. From a physiotherapy point of view you will be observing how much weight the patient is taking through his limbs and also noting his muscle tone, which may be normal, hypertonic or hypotonic.

Day 2

Continue with all the nursing care and physiotherapy from day 1, plus begin the following.

Passive range of motion exercises (PROM exercises) – are performed to maintain joint ROM. *N.B. Because the exercise is passive the patient does not receive any strengthening benefits from the PROM exercises.* If the patient has had cervical spinal surgery all four limbs may be affected; if surgery was in the thoracolumbar or lumbosacral region only his pelvic limbs will be affected.

When performing these exercises on the thoracic limbs the patient should be in lateral recumbency. Support the patient under the medial elbow with one hand to prevent any rotation of the joint and with the other hand bring all the joints together into full flexion. Then using the hand supporting the elbow to guide the movement, extend the joints in the thoracic limb; again avoid rotation by supporting the limb at the carpal joint. No *hold* is necessary at full flexion or extension. No pulling on the limb or tight gripping of the limb should occur. Three sets of 10 repetitions performed twice daily should be sufficient to maintain joint ROM (Figure 2.3; Video 2.1).

PROM exercises on the pelvic limbs follow the same formula as for the thoracic limbs, supporting at the medial stifle joint to prevent rotation(Figure 2.4; Video 2.2).

Stretches are important to maintain muscle length. If the patient is recumbent for a period of time muscle changes will occur resulting in muscle imbalance. If the flexors and internal rotator muscles become short and tight the patient will find it very difficult to ambulate even

VIDEO 2.1

Passive range of movement (PROM) exercises on a thoracic limb. A demonstration video of a home exercise programme that an owner can perform to maintain joint ROM.

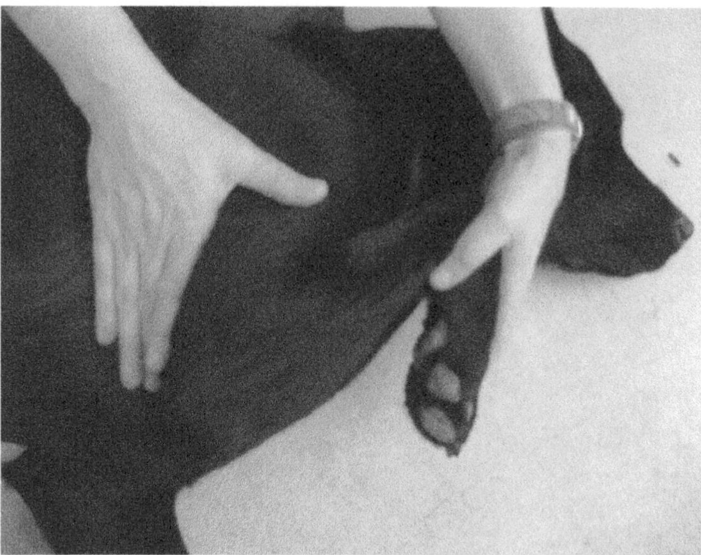

Figure 2.3 Right thoracic limb passive range of motion (PROM) exercise to maintain joint range of motion. The operator's right hand stabilises at the elbow joint to prevent rotation of the joint, the left hand flexes the carpal, elbow and shoulder joints.

VIDEO 2.2

Passive range of movement (PROM) exercises on a pelvic limb. A demonstration video of a home exercise programme that an owner can perform to maintain joint ROM.

with support as the limbs will be flexed and internally rotated, meaning he will not be able to place or position his feet and the limbs will be crossed over. It is easier to prevent muscle changes with stretching and positioning than it is to correct them.

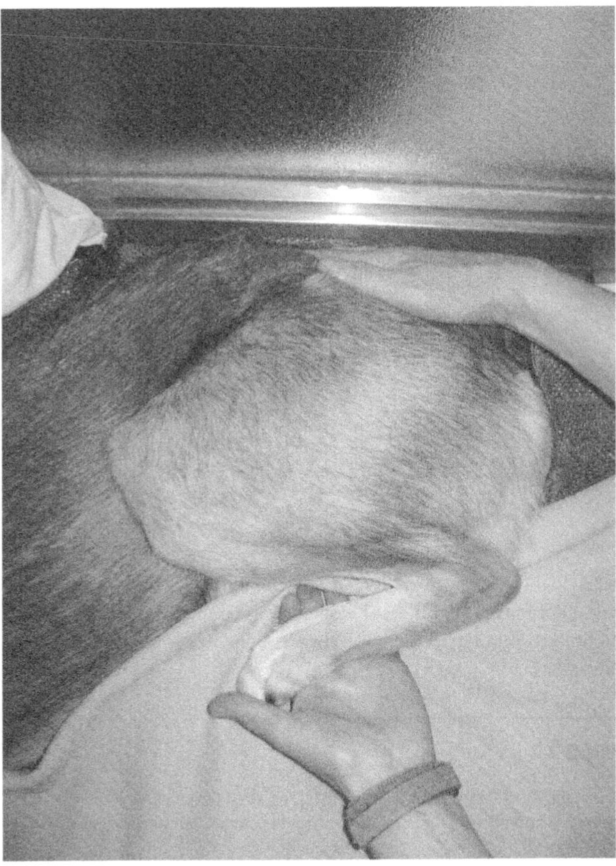

Figure 2.4 Left pelvic limb passive range of motion (PROM) exercise to maintain joint range of motion. The operator's right hand stabilises over the hip joint, the left hand flexes the tarsal, stifle and hip joints together.

Hip flexor stretch: The patient is placed in lateral recumbency with the limb to be stretched uppermost. One hand is placed at the level of the mid-femur, the other hand supports at the tarsal joint, and to avoid any rotation of the joints. The limb is passively extended until mild resistance is felt in the hip flexor muscle group (Figure 2.5). Stretches are held for 15 seconds, repeated three times, twice a day to maintain correct muscle length. Stretching should not be uncomfortable for the patient. *N.B. If the patient has undergone surgery in the lumbar spine region and has marked spinal flexion in this area, be gentle with this stretch as he may find it uncomfortable as extension of the hip will also extend the lumbar spine resulting in discomfort at the level of decompression.*

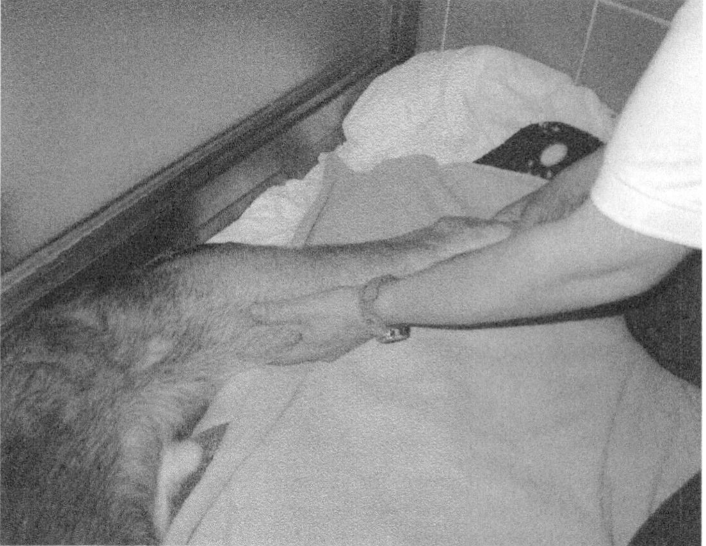

Figure 2.5 A left hip flexor stretch. The operator's left hand is placed on the distal femur and applies a caudal force into resistance; the right hand stabilises the distal limb to avoid any rotation of the joints.

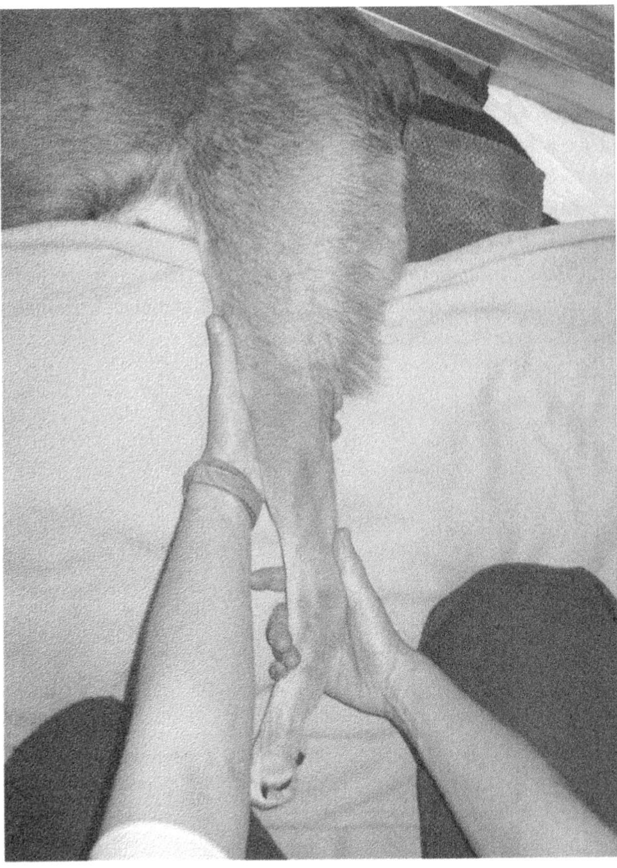

Figure 2.6 A left hamstring stretch. The operator's left hand is positioned on the distal femur and applies a caudal force; the right hand is positioned at the caudal tarsus and applies an opposing cranial force to stretch the hamstrings.

Hamstring stretch: Straighten the pelvic limb and place one hand at the level of the cranial mid-femur applying a caudally directed force, and place a second hand on the caudal aspect of the tarsal joint, applying an opposing cranially directed force (Figure 2.6). Stretches are held for 15 seconds, repeated three times, twice a day to maintain correct muscle length. Stretching should not be uncomfortable for the patient.

Adductor stretch: With the patient positioned in lateral recumbency flex the stifle to 90° support with one hand at the medial stifle then abduct the limb, position the other hand over the greater trochanter and apply a counter pressure to prevent any lax movement occurring at the hip joint. It may be useful to support the patient's lumbar sacral spine with your knee to prevent spinal rotation. Stretches are held for 15 seconds, repeated three times, twice a day to maintain correct muscle length. Stretching should not be uncomfortable for the patient (Video 2.3).

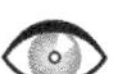

If the patient has undergone cervical spine surgery and the thoracic limbs are affected the triceps and internal rotators of the thoracic limbs should be stretched.

Triceps stretch: With the patient positioned in lateral recumbency place a hand on the caudal aspect of the elbow joint and advance the limb in a cranial direction until mild resistance is noted in the triceps. Use your other hand to support the limb at the carpal joint to avoid any rotation of the limb. Stretches are held for 15 seconds, repeated three times, twice a day to maintain correct muscle length. Stretching should not be uncomfortable for the patient (Figure 2.7; Video 2.4).

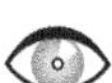

Internal rotator stretch: With the patient positioned in lateral recumbency use one hand to support the shoulder joint (humeral head), place your second hand on the medial aspect of the elbow joint and

VIDEO 2.3

Stretches for a pelvic limb. A demonstration video of a home exercise programme that an owner can perform to maintain muscle length.

VIDEO 2.4

Stretch for triceps muscle. A demonstration video of a home exercise programme that an owner can perform to maintain muscle length.

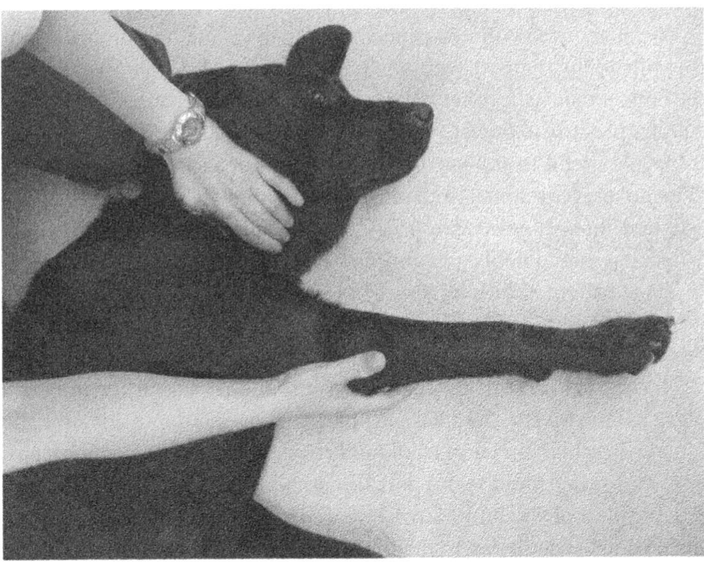

Figure 2.7 A right triceps stretch. The operator applies a cranial force to the caudal elbow into resistance to stretch the triceps muscle (see also Video 2.4).

rotate the limb externally to stretch the internal rotator muscle group. Stretches are held for 15 seconds, repeated three times, twice a day to maintain correct muscle length. Stretching should not be uncomfortable for the patient.

Biceps stretch: Caution is required when stretching the biceps if the patient has undergone ventral slot cervical spine surgery as this stretch may also stretch the surgical incision site.

N.B. If you or the surgeon have any concerns regarding this stretch then it may be better to omit this stretch.

With the patient positioned in lateral recumbency place one hand in the region of the mid-humerus, and apply a caudal force until mild resistance is noted in the biceps muscle; use a second hand to stabilise over the proximal humerus (Figure 2.8; Video 2.5) Stretches are held

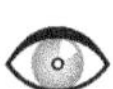

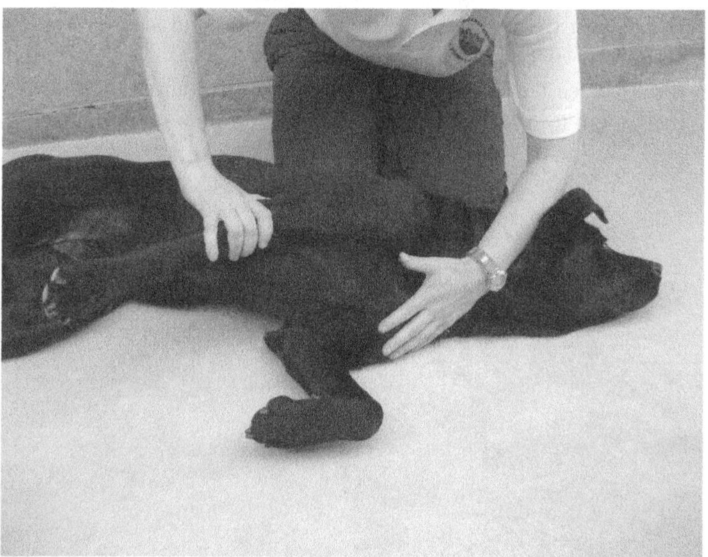

Figure 2.8 A right biceps stretch. The operator's left hand stabilises at the origin of the muscle, and the right hand is fixed on the insertion of the muscle and applies a caudal force into resistance to stretch the biceps.

VIDEO 2.5

Stretch for biceps muscle. A demonstration video of a home exercise programme that an owner can perform to maintain muscle length.

for 15 seconds, repeated three times, twice a day to maintain correct muscle length. Stretching should not be uncomfortable for the patient; avoid any rotation of the joints.

Following the passive exercises and with the veterinary surgeon's permission progress the supported standing exercises to supported gait practice. A minimum of two people will be required for this and ideally manual handling aids will be available to support the patient.

- Use a chest harness rather than a neck collar and lead, unless the lesion was very caudal.
- It may be easier to assist the patient from the kennel, then to step the patient into The Soft Quick Lift™ sling from a stable surface.

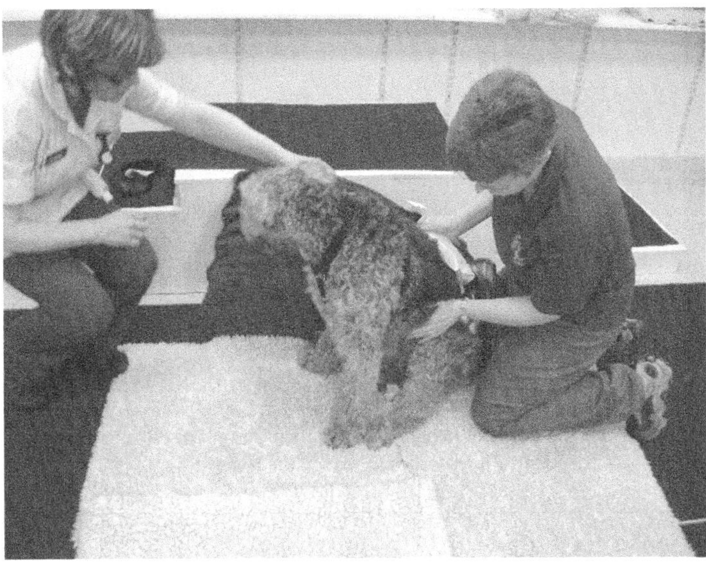

Figure 2.9 Assisted sitting in a paraparetic patient using The Soft Quick Lift™ sling. Note that the pelvic limbs are positioned in a functional sitting position, and the patient is being supported from behind to maintain his balance, and to prevent him from falling backwards.

- Use The Soft Quick Lift™ sling to assist the patient to ambulate (Figures 2.9 and 2.10); if the patient is mildly affected a Helping Hand sling maybe used.
- Use foot protectors as necessary.
- Ideally working as a team, each person should take one of The Soft Quick Lift™ handles. If the patient is very small one person can position themselves behind the patient and hold one of the handles in each hand.
- Aim to give the patient adequate support to facilitate *tip-toe* walking.
- Walk slowly and give the patient time to use the affected limbs.

The patient may be taken out two to three times daily for 2–5 minutes each time for toileting purposes. When the patient is returned

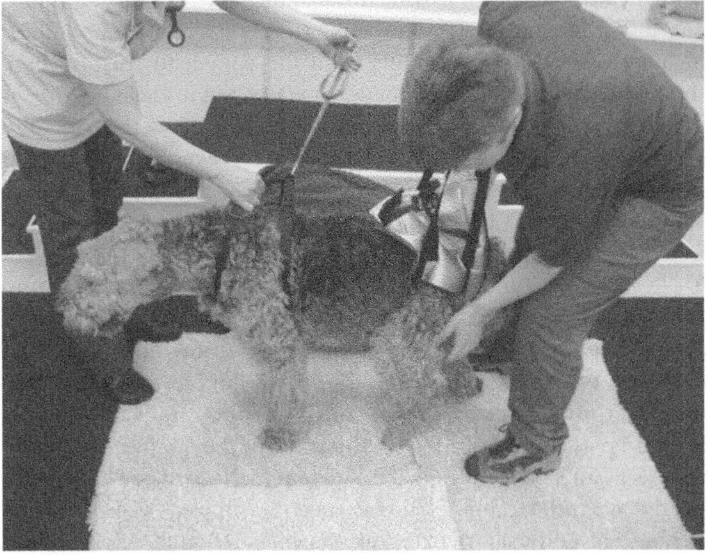

Figure 2.10 Assisted standing in a paraparetic patient using The Soft Quick Lift™ sling. Note the patient is taking some weight through the left pelvic limbs, but is knuckling on his right pelvic limb.

to his kennel ensure he is correctly positioned and supported to avoid muscle imbalances.

Days 3 and 4

Continue with the exercises from day 2.

Day 5

Hydrotherapy may commence on day 5 with the veterinary surgeon's permission. It is worth knowing beforehand if the patient is happy in water. If the patient is not happy in water and panics, the risks of the hydrotherapy may outweigh the benefits. Surgical sites can be protected with waterproof dressings.

Aims: Hydrotherapy can be used to increase the patient's buoyancy by reducing bodyweight passing through the limbs to facilitate voluntary motor function (VMF) in the limbs. It is essential that a trained member of staff is in the water with the patient to reassure him, should he panic, to support him in the water and to facilitate VMF in the affected limbs. Keep the first session short to allow the patient to become used to the exercise; 3 × 1 minutes of exercise with rests in between can be used as a starting guide. Begin with a slow speed to allow time for VMF in the affected limbs. The water should be comfortably warm at approximately 30°C.

Technique: An underwater treadmill (UWT) allows the patient to exercise in a functional way. Walking in the treadmill is a transferable activity to walking on dry land. Ensure at least two people are available, one in the water and one on dry land to control the settings and provide extra support to the patient. Buoyancy jackets should be available in a range of sizes; use the straps and clips to ensure a snug fit to utilise the buoyancy effect of the water. An overhead tracking hoist can be used to support large patients. A range of body slings, The Soft Quick Lift™ and Helping Hand slings should be available to support the patient in the hoist. This allows the person in the water to assist the patient to use his limbs in a functional way.

The buoyancy effect is relative to the amount of water supporting the patient. If the aim is to support the patient's weight and facilitate VMF a high level of buoyancy is required. However, care must be taken not to have the water too close to the patient's face as he may feel vulnerable, and the patient's feet should remain in contact with the treadmill belt and not float. A water level at the height of the patient's mid-trunk may be used as a starting guide. A slow speed should be selected, much slower than the patient's normal walking speed. This is to allow time for the patient to engage VMF in the affected limbs, which will be much slower than the motor function in the unaffected limbs. If the speed is too fast the patient will pull himself forwards with his unaffected limbs, and not allow time for weak early stage rehabilitation VMF in the affected limbs.

Patients may be discharged between days 5 and 10 postoperatively. This will depend on many factors such as how the patient has progressed with his mobility following surgery, if the patient has independent bladder function, the owner's home situation, and their ability to assist the patient to maximum recovery and function.

No two patients are the same – even if they have undergone the same procedure their recovery rates will vary. Some patients may have concurrent joint disease, which will affect their rehabilitation. It is important that patients who are on medication for joint disease continue this medication while hospitalised.

Bladder function may be altered in neurological patients with spinal cord compression. Following spinal decompression bladder control may still be compromised and the patient's bladder should be palpated every 4–6 hours to assess size and to monitor how firm the bladder is. If in any doubt bladder size can be confirmed with a quick ultrasound scan. If the bladder becomes large and firm and the patient does not empty the bladder himself it may need to be manually expressed, or catheterised. When the patient begins to regain bladder control the flow may be weaker so it is important to provide him with time and support to empty his bladder.

If access to the owner's house has steps, and the patient is too heavy for the owner to carry, the rehabilitation programme in the hospital may need to include stair practice. This will require two people, one to lead the patient and a second to support the patient with The Soft Quick Lift™ sling or a Helping Hand sling on the stairs. The patient will need support ascending the stairs as he will have reduced strength to push off on the pelvic limbs, and his balance will be affected on the descent so he will require close support to maintain his balance.

At the time of discharge the owner is provided with a progressive rehabilitation programme to assist the patient back to his highest level of function. Spend time demonstrating the exercises to the owner and allow the owner time to practise the exercises under supervision. Show the owner how to use any slings and foot protectors the patient may be discharged with. Ensure the owner gives the patient adequate support when using slings to ensure the patient does not damage his feet on rough surfaces, but ensure that the owner does not *carry* the pelvic limbs for the patient. Ask the owner to aim for *tip toe* walking support and ensure the patient walks slowly to allow VMF in the affected limbs. Finally, show the owner how to lift the patient in and out of the car. Under no circumstances should the patient be allowed to jump in or out of the car. Small dogs can be lifted by one person supporting the animal with one hand under the abdomen and a second hand in front of the chest. Larger dogs should be lifted by two people, with one supporting the animal under the chest and a second person supporting him under the abdomen; when lowering the patient place his unaffected limbs onto the stable surface just ahead of his affected limbs so he can take his weight in a controlled manner.

Physiotherapy home exercise programme following hemi-laminectomy for IVDD T13 - L1

Early phase (approx. 0–2 weeks)

Passive range of motion (PROM) exercises

Flex the joints in the hind limbs, and then extend the joints.
Repeat three sets of 10 repetitions.

Mobility

Gentle controlled walking with sling support on a flat, firm, non-slip surfaces, 5 minutes, four times a day. Try to ensure the patient does not scuff his toes on hard surfaces; use foot protectors as necessary.

Stretches

Stretch hamstrings, and a *gentle* hip flexor muscle stretch twice daily; hold each stretch for 15 seconds, and repeat three times.

Positioning

Place a small pillow or folded towel between the back legs if the patient is lying on his side for long periods of time.

Sitting and standing practice

Try to encourage the patient to spend some of his day sitting and standing; give him only the support that is necessary and ensure his back feet are positioned correctly.

Mid-phase (approx. 2–4 weeks)

Mobility

Start to add into the exercise plan work on gentle slopes up and down, and weaving between objects, 5 minutes, four times a day. The patient may not need the sling support at this stage; however, if he is still weak or unable to maintain his standing balance continue to use the sling.

Strengthening

Sit to stand exercises, two sets of 5 repetitions; assist the patient only as necessary.

Balance

To improve the patient's standing balance, gently nudge him at the hips right to left side, then left to right.

Continue with the exercises from the early phase.

Late phase (approx. 4–6 weeks)

Mobility

Continue with mobility as in mid-phase; add in stepping over small logs or rolls and increase duration of walks to 10–15 minutes, four times a day. Also begin to exercise the patient on different surfaces, for example concrete, grass, bark chippings and sand.

Continue with the exercises from the mid phase.

Don'ts

Do not allow the patient to jump on/off furniture or in and out of cars, or to play vigorously with other animals while he is recovering. He may be unsteady on stairs; if so do not allow him on the stairs. When he is not being supervised he should be kept in a confined area so he does not try to do too much and possibly injure himself.

Follow-up outpatient physiotherapy

Follow-up physiotherapy should be offered to clients to maximise patient recovery and function. If the patient is not local to your area referral to a facility closer to the owner's home may be required. Patients are usually seen once a week following discharge to facilitate VMF and improve strength, balance, proprioception and stamina.

Weaving cones can be used to improve weight transfer on the affected limbs and challenge balance. Begin with the cones at least as far apart as the patient's body as lateral spinal flexion may not be comfortable for the patient in the early stages.

Cavaletti poles can be used to encourage joint flexion and paw placement. Be aware that as the patient regains function in his limbs proximal joint movements will be greater than distal joint movements so hip flexion will be stronger than tarsal dorsiflexion and the patient may knuckle on his pelvic limbs for some time following surgery. Use slings and foot protectors as necessary to support the patient (Video 2.6).

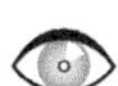

Laser treatment over the surgical site can be used weekly to reduce inflammation and counter excessive fibrous tissue formation, and to improve nerve cell amplitude to increase muscle action. Power settings and duration of treatment will be determined by species, skin colour, weight, the area to be treated, and the stage of the condition (acute or chronic). Select chronic at this stage.

Unless the patient has stairs in the house, stair practice should not begin until 4 weeks postoperatively; stair climbing requires a high level of motor function, strength and balance. The spine will be in extension on the stairs and this may be uncomfortable for patients who have had surgery in the lumbar spine region.

Peanut balls should be used with caution in surgical spinal patients to prevent injury to the surgical area. Wobble boards are not recommended for at least 6 weeks following spinal surgery as any jerky uncontrolled movements may have an adverse affect on the recent spinal surgery.

VIDEO 2.6

Outpatient exercises. (a) Weaving: the patient shows reduced spinal flexion as she steps between the cones then turns. She is also weak/paretic on pelvic limbs with reduced balance. (b) Cavaletti poles: the patient is reluctant to begin with, and then shows good pelvic limb proprioception. (c) Stairs: the patient is weak (crouched pelvic limb gait) on ascent, but has good balance on descent.

Hydrotherapy using a UWT can be used to facilitate VMF and strengthen the weak affected limbs, to improve core stability, and increase joint ROM. The speed of the belt can be controlled to allow extra time for motor function in the weak affected limbs. As the patient progresses the speed of the belt can be increased to improve stamina, and resistance can also be added to improve strength. The temperature of the water can be adjusted for patient comfort. The height of the water can be adjusted; buoyancy may be desirable in early to mid stages of rehabilitation. However, as the patient progresses the water can be used to provide resistance and strengthen muscles. Most resistance is found at the surface level of the water, so set the level of the water to match the muscle group you wish to strengthen; for example, water at the level of mid-femur will strengthen the quadriceps and hamstrings muscle groups (Video 2.7).

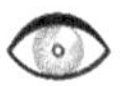

Outcome measures

Objective outcome measures are useful tools to establish baseline performance data, and to measure patient progress. Baseline outcome measures may also guide goal setting to improve patient performance. Outcome measures can be used to evaluate patient progress: usually re-measure at 6 weeks and compare with baseline measures, then measure outcomes again at 12 weeks, and compare against 6 weeks' outcome measures.

Gait – can be recorded on a digital camera and subsequent recordings can be made over time to monitor progress. Baseline measures may well show the patient to be non-ambulatory and mobilising with a sling and assistance. Subsequent recordings may show the patient

VIDEO 2.7

Outpatient hydrotherapy. The patient has an ataxic pelvic limb gait (high-stepping gait pattern), with wide pelvic limb stance to maintain balance.

has progressed to weak ambulatory status, with pelvic limb ataxia. At the time of discharge from outpatient physiotherapy the patient may still have mild neurological balance and proprioception deficits, but will have hopefully progressed to a functionally independent status.

Posture – may be altered in spinal patients. A kyphotic or flexed thoracolumbar spine is common following surgery of the spine in this area. Over time and with adequate pain control, pain and inflammation will subside and the patient will begin to relax tense muscles. Walking will gently extend the thoraco-lumbar spine therefore further reducing spinal flexion.

If spinal posture remains problematic 4–6 weeks post-surgery and the patient is not uncomfortable, careful spinal mobilisations may be carried out by a physiotherapist to improve spinal posture.

Patients who have undergone ventral slot surgery may have a slightly low head carriage or reduced cervical spine extension. These patients usually have functional ROM in the cervical spine and slightly reduced cervical spine extension will not affect their quality of life.

Muscle mass – animals with a degree of spinal cord compression will show muscle mass reduction and weakness in the associated limbs. If the lesion is in the cervical spine all four limbs may be affected; if the lesion is in the thoraco-lumbar, or lumbo-sacral region only the pelvic limbs will be affected. Objectively muscle mass should be measured using a tape measure around the circumference of the muscle belly, as this is where changes in muscle mass are most apparent. Ensure consistency so if the patient was measured in lying ensure this same position is adopted each time the patient is measured. It is good practice to take three measures of the circumference of the limb at the level of the muscle belly then use the average from these readings to record muscle mass.

Remember that in Hansen type II disc disease the patient may have been deteriorating slowly over a period of time so may have marked muscle mass reduction, and weakness in the affected limbs. Immediately following surgical intervention it is not unusual for patients to deteriorate further, before they begin to slowly progress. Muscle strengthening programmes usually follow a 6-week programme so this would be the time to measure and compare results with the initial baseline measure to record any changes in muscle mass.

Weight-bearing status – directly relates to function. If the animal is not distributing weight equally through the limbs he will be overloading the non-affected limbs, which can lead to secondary complications from the extra stress placed on those joints. Strength is also related to weight-bearing; if the animal is not weight-bearing through the limbs normally the affected limbs will lose muscle mass and strength.

Weight-bearing status is best observed in stance, when it may be obvious the patient is shifting his weight onto the unaffected limbs. He may stand with the affected limb(s) slightly flexed if weak (paretic), or he may hold the affected limb towards his mid-line to off load the weight and to aid his balance. Observation of the paws in stance may give an indication of weight passing through the limbs. The paws of the limbs that are taking additional bodyweight may appear slightly splayed when compared to the paw(s) of the affected limb. Supporting the patient and lifting the affected limb(s) will give an indication of the weight passing through the limbs. The affected limbs will be easier to lift as the animal's weight-bearing status is reduced compared to limb lifting in the unaffected limbs. When an unaffected limb is lifted the animal may sink on the affected limb as this will be subject to extra weight-bearing.

Normal bathroom weighing scales have been shown to be effective in measuring weight-bearing status in animals. Pressure-sensitive mats will also objectively measure weight-bearing status through the limbs. It is worth noting that many pressure-sensitive mats are manufactured for the human market and as such all four of the animal's feet cannot be placed on the mat at the same time (human pressure mats are designed to measure two pressure points only). Since an animal may shift his weight onto the contralateral limb or diagonally contralaterally it is good practice to measure and compare:

The pelvic limbs then the thoracic limbs. If unaffected, the distribution of weight will be equal, that is, 50% on each limb. Measure left hemi-limbs then right hemi-limbs; if unaffected the distribution of weight will be 60% in the thoracic limb and 40% in the pelvic limb. It is good practice to measure three times and then take an average reading to record weight-bearing status through the limbs.

Conscious proprioception – this test can be carried out on all four limbs in turn to assess the animal's awareness of joint position. The animal stands squarely and is supported as necessary by the assessor. The limb to be assessed is turned over by the assessor so the animal is weight-bearing or 'knuckling' on the dorsal surface of the limb. It is usual for the assessor to repeat the test three times. The normal response is for the animal to correct the paw position immediately. The response can be classified as present (normal), delayed or absent. In the pelvic limb this test would assess conscious proprioception in the tarsal joint; in the thoracic limb the test would assess conscious proprioception in the carpal joint.

A paper test can also be used to assess conscious proprioception in the proximal limb joints. The limb to be tested is placed on a thick sheet of paper; the paper is then gentle withdrawn in a caudal direction. The normal response for the animal is to step off the sheet of paper and to bring the limb forwards.

Cervical spondylomyelopathy (wobbler syndrome)

This condition is the result of congenital and degenerative changes involving compression of the cervical spinal cord. Large breeds such as great Danes and Dobermans are typically affected. Clinical signs may include neck pain, ataxia and tetraparesis.

Medical management may be considered for mild cases; however, since this is a degenerative condition surgery may be required at a later stage. The aim of surgery is to decompress and stabilise the cervical spine.

Spinal column fractures or dislocations

Fractures and dislocations of the spinal column occur most often secondary to external trauma. The thoraco-lumbar region is the most commonly affected site. High-speed impact injuries, such as when a greyhound chases a rabbit then collides with a tree, may result in cervical spine fracture-dislocation. Within the cervical spine region the atlanto-axial junction is considered a weak area as it relies on ligaments for stability. Medical management with analgesia, cage rest and placement of an external splint may be considered in cases with mild neurological deficits, without spinal compression and minimally displaced fractures or luxations.

Surgical management involving open reduction and internal fixation would be indicated for treatment of spinal cord compression, or in cases of vertebral instability with severe neurological deficits.

Non-surgical presenting conditions

Fibrocartilaginous embolism

Fibrocartilaginous embolism (FCE) occurs when a fragment of fibrocartilage from an intervertebral disc breaks away and becomes lodged in the spinal cord vasculature causing an embolism resulting in ischaemic necrosis of the spinal cord grey matter (Cauzinille & Kornegay, 1996). The condition is sometimes referred to as an ischaemic myelopathy (Figure 2.11).

Onset of clinical signs is sudden, and may be associated with vigorous exercise such as jumping and twisting awkwardly to catch a ball. Lesions are often lateralised and non-painful. Magnetic resonance imaging (MRI) demonstrates an area of intramedullary hyperintensity in the region of the infarct. Improvement can be dramatic in the early stage and continues at a slower rate over many months. Early intervention with physiotherapy has been shown to aid recovery.

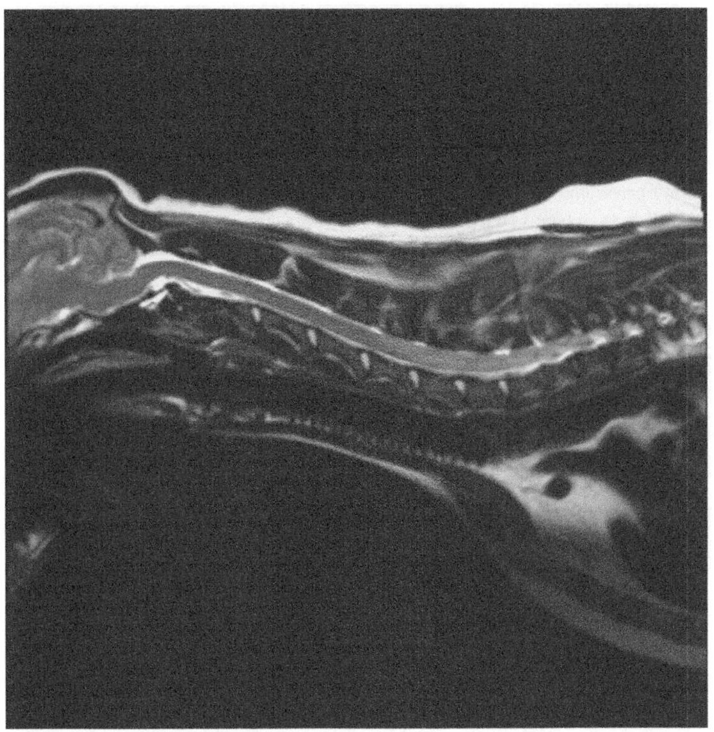

Figure 2.11 The image shows a suspected C6-7 fibrocartilaginous embolism (FCE) lesion.

As for most spinal cord injuries physiotherapy is recommended to rehabilitate the animal back to its highest level of function (Gandini et al., 2003) (Videos 2.8 and 2.9).

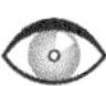

Type III disc disease

Type III disc disease may also be referred to as a *traumatic non-compressive disc lesion,* or as an *acute non-compressive nucleus pulposus extrusion.* It occurs when healthy disc material extrudes through the

VIDEO 2.8

Fibrocartilaginous embolism (FCE) gait, no rehabilitation. The patient suffered a FCE and did not receive any formal rehabilitation as it was not available at that time (7 years ago). Note the over-developed musculature of the thoracic limbs, and muscle atrophy of the pelvic limbs. The patient is weakest on the left pelvic limb, which gives way on her. The patient also shows reduced balance and poor spinal posture.

VIDEO 2.9

Fibrocartilaginous embolism (FCE) gait in a dog using a Walkin' Wheels® device (Wheels4dogs, Penzance, Cornwall, UK). Note the patient is still using her pelvic limbs and shows an improved gait pattern with increased joint range of motion (ROM), stride length, balance and spinal posture. The Walkin' Wheels® provides the patient with stability and allows her to go for longer walks and so enhances her quality of life.

annulus hitting the spinal cord at speed causing a considerable concussive impact on the cord. The gel-like disc material immediately disperses, leaving no resultant compression (Yarrow & Jeffery, 2000). Type III disc disease is often seen in young animals following vigorous activity.

Contusion of the spinal cord results in impairment of the perfusion of the affected area of the cord as the vessels supplying the spine are damaged. The system of autoregulation of spinal blood pressure is also impaired, further exacerbating damage to the spine (Tator & Fehlings, 1991). Subsequently, a complex cascade of biochemical changes is triggered, beginning within moments of the injury but peaking at 2–4 days after the initial insult, causing neuronal cell death and inflammatory reaction (Jeffery & Blakemore, 1999).

CASE STUDY: PHYSIOTHERAPY REHABILITATION PROGRAMME FOR A TRAUMATIC DISC (TYPE III DISC)

Clinical history

Sam is a 2-year-old male labradoodle. He presented for investigation of acute onset of non-ambulatory tetraparesis progressing over 12 hours. He was found unable to stand the evening prior to presentation but still had voluntary movements in all four limbs, stronger in the thoracic limbs. The next day he had lost voluntary movement and pain perception in the right thoracic limb.

General examination was unremarkable. Weight: 27.9 kg; temperature: 37.6°C; pulse: 64 bpm; respiratory rate: 20 bpm.

Neurological examination

- *Mentation*: normal.
- *Gait*: non-ambulatory tetraparesis, with plegia in the right thoracic limb, and both pelvic limbs. Good voluntary movements present in the left thoracic limb. Deep pain perception was absent in the right thoracic limb, but present in both pelvic limbs.
- *Conscious proprioception*: absent right thoracic limb, and both pelvic limbs, and delayed in the left thoracic limb.
- *Segmental reflexes*: delayed withdrawal left thoracic limb, absent right thoracic limb, normal both pelvic limbs.
- *Cutaneous trunci*: sluggish throughout (worse on right side).
- *Cranial nerves*: bilateral Horner's syndrome (worse on right side). No obvious spinal pain.
- *Localisation*: based on the neurological examination the lesion was localised to C6-T2 spinal segments.

Investigations

- Routine biochemistry and haematology were unremarkable.
- MRI of the cervical spine showed a right-sided intramedullary hyperintensity from C5-6 to caudal C7, more central at the level of C6-7, associated with cord swelling (Figure 2.12). There was also a dehydrated disc at C6-7

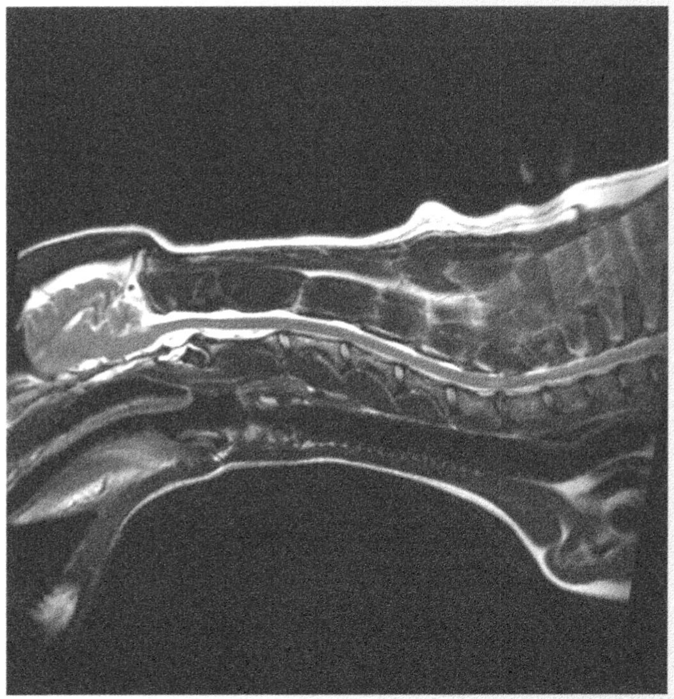

Figure 2.12 The image shows a right-sided intramedullary hyperintensity from C5-6 to caudal C7, more central at the level of C7, associated with cord swelling. These features are consistent with a type III disc at C6-7.

and mild disc protrusion, suggestive of mild chronic degenerative changes. These features are consistent with a traumatic disc at C6-7 or ischaemic infarction (FCE).

- Cerebrospinal fluid (CSF) analysis (lumbar puncture) was unremarkable.

Diagnosis

Suspected traumatic disc C6-7

Inpatient treatment

Sam was hospitalised and an indwelling urinary catheter placed.

Physiotherapy

Physiotherapy and rehabilitation for non-surgical spinal trauma cases, typically type III traumatic discs and FCE, begin early and tend to be more vigorous as no surgery has taken place and the aim is to rehabilitate the patient back to his highest level of function as quickly as possible. An animal on strict cage rest will develop secondary joint and muscle changes.

Non-surgical patients can present similar to surgical patients. With paresis or paralysis of the affected limbs, changes in conscious proprioception (CP), ataxia and altered bladder control are common to both surgical and non-surgical spinal trauma cases. The prognosis for recovery in non-surgical cases is difficult to make; early progress is usually seen as a good indicator of a favourable prognosis. However, animals can make a remarkable recovery even when progress is very slow initially.

Secondary changes in joints and muscles must be prevented. PROM exercises will maintain joint ROM and reduce inflammation. Stretches and positioning will prevent muscle changes and imbalances. These exercises should commence on day 1 and be performed at least twice daily as a minimum requirement to prevent secondary changes.

Laser therapy, if available, can commence daily from day 1. Treatment should include the area over the spinal lesion; extend treatment to include four disc spaces cranial and four disc spaces caudal to the site of the lesion. Biochemical changes associated with the trauma and inflammation will reach a peak between days 2 and 4 post-injury. These biochemical changes result in oedema, which usually extends caudal to the lesion. Because of these changes the patient can deteriorate further in the early days following the initial trauma. By commencing early laser treatment to the affected area the aim is to reduce inflammation, oedema and pain (if present), and improve vascular activity and nerve function. Laser light causes vasodilation, increasing blood flow to the affected area to improve healing, and speeding up nerve cell reconnection thereby increasing nerve conduction velocity and muscle activity, resulting in a more favourable outcome for the patient.

The physiotherapy exercise programme is progressive so day 1 exercises should be carried forwards to day 2, then both day 1 and 2 exercises should be carried over to day 3 and so on.

Day 2 will build on the exercises from day 1. Begin standing exercises and gait practice using appropriate aids and protection of the affected distal limbs as necessary.

If by day 3 the patient has progressed sufficiently and has VMF in the affected limb(s) but not placement of the limbs, weight-bearing exercises over a peanut ball can commence to encourage weight-bearing through the affected limbs. Two people will be required for this to ensure the patient feels secure and does not panic.

Aims: Weight-bearing over the peanut utilises extensor muscle activity in the limbs and encourages correct placement of the feet. It also supports the patient's trunk so he does not need to support all of his own weight; because it is an unstable surface the patient will also engage postural and core stability muscles to maintain balance on the peanut ball. Good postural muscle control is essential for standing and static balance. Core stability is essential for dynamic balance and to control pelvic postural sway. Poor core stability can contribute to altered joint biomechanics and increases stress on the spinal column, which could lead to stiffness and arthritis in the spine resulting in reduced flexibility and mobility.

Technique: The patient is supported at the trunk by one person and a second person supports the patient at the pelvis. Together they lift the patient onto the peanut with his limbs just touching or just off the ground. The first person should support the patient at the shoulders. It is important to keep in close to the patient so he feels secure and does not panic. If the patient has a lesion in the cervical spine area it may be necessary for the first person to also support the weight of the patient's head.

The second person supports the patient at the pelvis and the patient is gently rocked forwards and backwards to encourage weight-bearing through the limbs. If the patient *knuckles* on any limb, passively correct his paw position. Rocking the patient gently side to side can target weight-bearing towards a weaker limb in monoparetic patients.

Keep the session short and allow the patient time to become used to the exercise. If the patient panics and will not settle with assurance, as a team carefully remove him from the peanut. The benefits of the exercise are not worth the risks if he falls or twists awkwardly.

Cautions: Do not allow the patient to stand on the peanut, this is a very advanced balancing activity and not suitable for a patient recovering from major spinal trauma. *Do not attempt to manage a patient on the peanut ball alone – a minimum of two people will be required for patient safety.*

If the patient is happy in water, hydrotherapy using a UWT could also commence. Keep the session short to begin with, provide the patient with plenty of rest breaks, and use the water to provide buoyancy and facilitate VMF in the affected limb(s). Also continue with day 1 and 2 exercises.

If the patient continues to progress, active-assisted exercises can also commence on day 4. Active-assisted exercises (using slings as necessary) aim to maximise the patient's potential. While the patient may not be at a level where he can actively exercise independently he may have recovered sufficient VMF and strength in the affected limbs so that with assistance he is able to exercise. Weaving cones spaced at a distance greater than the animal's body length can be used to encourage weight transfer and adduction and abduction of the affected limbs. This exercise is also useful for early balance rehabilitation and encourages lateral spinal flexion. Cavaletti poles at a low height (approximately 5 cm) can be used to encourage the patient to flex his affected limbs and also the visual prompt may encourage him to think about where he is placing the affected limbs and so facilitate improvements in CP. Continue with all the previous day's exercises.

Assuming the patient continues to progress and working towards his imminent discharge, begin to increase the duration of his active-assisted exercises and reduce the support given to him if appropriate, to build his stamina. If the patient has stairs at home that he needs to be able to manage, begin stair practice work. Remember this will require two people to ensure the patient is safe on the stairs.

Early balance work may commence using wobble cushions as an unstable surface under the affected limb. Start by placing a single wobble cushion under the patient's affected limb; ensure the patient has adequate support and is not *knuckling* on the limb. Once the patient is confident standing on the unstable surface, gently nudge him at the contralateral hip so he is taking extra weight through the affected limb. Progress by placing a second affected limb on a second wobble cushion; aim to give the patient only the support he requires to maintain his balance. This exercise can be progressed further by incorporating single limb lifting, with the affected limb on the wobble cushion. This exercise will challenge balance, strength and core stability.

Prior to discharge it is often desirable to arrange for the owner to join in with a physiotherapy session. The patient often finds the presence of his owner to be motivating, and makes extra effort in the owner's presence. During this session the owner can observe the passive and active-assisted exercises the patient is working on and it is also an ideal opportunity for the owner to practice the passive and active-assisted exercises under supervision as they will be required to carry out the exercises at home once the patient is discharged. Ideally the patient will continue with formal weekly physiotherapy appointments until he plateaus to maximise his return to function and quality of life.

Physiotherapy rehabilitation home exercise programme following C6-7 traumatic disc

Early phase (approx. 0–3 weeks)

Passive range of motion (PROM) exercises: Passively flex the joints in the pelvic limbs, and then extend the joints. Repeat the flexion and extension exercises in the thoracic limbs. Three sets of 10 repetitions per limb.

- *Mobility:* Gentle controlled walking with a harness and sling support as necessary on flat, firm surfaces, 5 minutes, four times daily. Try to ensure the patient does not scuff his toes on hard surfaces. Stay on his left side (he is weaker on his right side).
- *Stretches:* Stretch hamstrings, hip flexor, biceps and triceps muscles; hold each stretch for 15 seconds, repeat each stretch three times, twice a day.
- *Positioning:* Place a small pillow or folded towel between the thoracic and pelvic limbs if the patient is lying on his side for a long period of time. If possible it is preferable for his chest to be positioned in sternal recumbency, with his head supported in neutral, and his left hip positioned down, then turn his hips every 4 hours. (If he is unable to change his own position, and turn himself).
- *Sitting and standing practice:* Try to encourage the patient to spend some of his day sitting and standing; give him only the minimal support when he is standing and ensure all four feet are positioned correctly. Stay on his left side.

Mid-phase (approx. weeks 3–6)

Mobility: Start to add gentle slopes up and down and weaving between objects into the exercise plan: 5 minutes, four times a day.

- *Strengthening:* Sit to stand exercises, two sets of 5 repetitions; assist the patient only as necessary.

- *Balance:* The patient's balance reactions are reduced. Improve his standing balance by gently nudging him at the hips left to right side, then right to left. Repeat at the shoulder, nudging left to right side, then right to left.
- Continue with exercises as in early phase.

Late phase (approx. weeks 6–9)

Mobility: Continue with mobility as in mid-phase; add in stepping over small logs or rolls and increase duration to 10–15 minutes four times daily. Also begin to exercise the patient on different surfaces, for example concrete, grass, bark chippings and sand.

- Continue with the exercises from mid phase.

Don'ts

Do not allow the patient to go up or down stairs, jump on/off furniture or in/out of cars or to play vigorously with other dogs until he is checked by the veterinary surgeon in 4 weeks time. Keep him restricted to a small area when he is not being closely supervised so he does not fall and injure himself.

Outpatient physiotherapy or onward referral

Ideally patients should be seen as outpatients once a week following discharge. The aims of the programme will be to improve strength, balance, proprioception, functional activities and stamina, using hydrotherapy, weaving cones, balance boards, cavaletti poles and stairs.

Medical neurological presenting conditions

Acute polyradiculoneuritis

Acute polyradiculoneuritis is caused by an inflammatory reaction of the axons and myelin sheaths, which is most intense at the level of the ventral nerve root (Cummings & Haas, 1966). The disease can be classified according to cause as:

1 Coonhound paralysis (seen in North America after racoon bites).
2 Idiopathic polyradicular neuritis.
3 Post-vaccine polyradicular neuritis (extremely rare).

A recent study has shown that dogs with idiopathic acute polyradicular neuritis are more likely to have positive titres for *Toxoplasma gondii* than control dogs (Holt et al., 2011).

Clinical signs

1 Lower motor neuron (LMN) tetraparesis or tetraplegia.
2 Dysphonia and facial weakness.
3 Respiratory compromise in extreme cases.

Diagnosis

1 A presumptive diagnosis is based on the presentation of clinical signs – a limited number of diseases cause acute-onset LMN tetraparesis/tetraplegia.
2 Electromyography (EMG) reveals spontaneous electrical activity consistent with denervation.
3 Nerve biopsy provides a definitive diagnosis.

Treatment

Take into consideration the patient's mental status and anxiety levels and provide support as necessary. The patient may also require assistance to eat and drink.

If hypoventilation is suspected, arterial blood gas analysis should be performed to determine if mechanical ventilation is necessary. If blood gas analysis is not immediately available, pulse oximetry can be used to measure oxygen saturation (SPO_2) these measures will give an indication of the patient's oxygen exchange status.

Physiotherapy

- Passive range of motion (PROM) exercises of the affected limbs to maintain joint range of motion (three sets of 10 repetitions, 2–3 times a day).

- Protraction, retraction and internal rotator stretches of the affected limbs to maintain muscle length and prevent muscle contractions (three stretches with a 15 second hold for each stretch, repeat 2–3 times daily).
- Monitor respiratory rate, effort and measure SPO_2 to ensure adequate oxygenation.
- Sitting practice to encourage weight-bearing through the thoracic limbs; support the patient's trunk as necessary.
- Supported standing: use a *peanut*-type physio ball to support bodyweight or a *body sling.*
- Gait practice using slings and hoists if available; walk slowly to allow time for movement in the affected limbs. Aim for toe touching weight-bearing exercise providing the patient with plenty of support as he will be too weak to support his own bodyweight. Aim for little and often to begin with as the patient will fatigue quickly. *Quality* rather than *quantity* of movement is desirable in the early stages of recovery. *He may also need to have his head supported when walking in the early stages.*
- If the patient is unable to turn himself he should be turned from left to right sides every 4 hours; positioning aids such as wedges should be placed between his thoracic and pelvic limbs to maintain them in a neutral position, and to minimise muscle imbalances between internal and external rotators. Internal rotators tend to become short and tight, and external rotators tend to become long and weak. Alternatively, position the trunk in sternal recumbency and support the head in a neutral position with a wedge; this position is preferred to maximise respiratory gaseous exchange in recumbent patients. The hips can be turned to left or right sides every 4 hours, with an adductor wedge placed between the hips to support them in a neutral position, with the aim of preventing muscle imbalance. Protect the elbows and all bony prominences; ideally use a waterproof mattress covered with vetbed®.

As the patient progresses he will require less support; aim to increase his strength, stamina and balance.

Tetanus

Tetanus is a diffuse neuromuscular toxic disease caused by absorption of tetanus toxin, *tetanospasmin*, produced by the anaerobic bacterium *Clostridium tetani*. The toxin is absorbed into the bloodstream and from there is taken up by the nerves.

Tetanospasmin has zinc metalloproteinease activity and binds to and clears synaptobrevin preventing the release of neurotransmitter (Binz et al., 2010).

Clinical signs

1 Generalised increase in extensor tone demonstrated as a stiff gait pattern, raised tail, increased facial tone, rigid ears, miotic pupils, lips drawn back, forehead wrinkled, profuse salivation and difficulty swallowing.
2 Visual and tactile stimulation may further increase the animal's muscle tone, and lead to muscle spasm.
3 Symptoms may progress to include respiratory compromise and mega-oesophagus as a result of increased diaphragmatic tone.

Diagnosis

A tetanus diagnosis may be presumptive based on clinical signs; the presence of a wound or recent surgery would further support the diagnosis.

Treatment

- Antibiotics.
- Debridement and flushing of the wound with hydrogen peroxide.
- Diazepam to reduce extensor tone.
- Reduce visual and tactile stimuli.
- Consider placing a gastrotomy tube (if severe mega-oesophagus).

- Consider placing a tracheostomy tube (if respiratory compromise).
- Consider bladder catheterisation.

Physiotherapy

- Massage of the affected muscle to reduce high tone.
- PROM exercises to break up high tone.
- Stretch biceps and hamstrings muscle groups.
- Monitor respiratory function; provide percussion (coupage) if indicated (if the patient is retaining secretions).
- Supported standing exercises to maintain muscle length and strength.
- Supported gait practice on non-slip floors using slings to support the patient as necessary.
- Position the patient in sternal recumbency, as he may not tolerate lateral recumbency and regular turning.

Myasthenia gravis

Immune-mediated myasthenia gravis is a relatively common neuromuscular disease affecting dogs and occasionally cats (Shelton, 2002).

Myasthenia gravis is characterised by failure of neuromuscular transmission due to the reduction in the number of functional nicotinic acetylcholine receptors on the postsynaptic membrane of the neuromuscular junction. This deficiency of functional receptors reduces the sensitivity of the postsynaptic membrane to acetylcholine (Shelton, 2002).

Clinical signs

- Facial paresis.
- Regurgitation.
- Mega-oesophagus.
- Dysphagia.
- Severe exercise intolerance.
- Paralysis.

Diagnosis

A presumptive diagnosis of myasthenia gravis may be made following the resolution of muscle weakness as a result of an injection of edrophonium chloride (Tensilon test). This can be confirmed with a positive acetylcholine receptor antibody titre.

Treatment

- Anticholinesterase drugs.
- If poor response to the above, a low-dose corticosteroid may be considered (if there is no evidence of aspiration pneumonia present).

Supportive care

- Elevation of food and water bowls.
- Hand feed food shaped into small meatballs while maintaining the animal in an upright position to encourage food to pass into the stomach.
- Consider placing a percutaneous endoscopic gastrotomy tube (PEG) if mega-oesophagus and aspiration pneumonia are present.

Physiotherapy

- PROM exercises to maintain joint range; patients tend to be low tone so three sets of 10 repetitions twice daily is sufficient.
- Stretch biceps, triceps, internal rotators, hip flexors, hamstrings and adductors three times; hold each stretch for 15 seconds and repeat twice daily.
- Monitor respiratory function; provide percussion (coupage) as indicated.
- Standing and gait practice with assistance and slings as necessary to maintain strength and encourage clearance of chest secretions (do this before feeding, to reduce the risk of regurgitation and aspiration).
- The patient may prefer to rest in sternal rather than lateral recumbency. In sternal recumbency he will have improved oxygen exchange and is able to cough and clear secretions.

- He may benefit from having a raised pad to rest his head on and reduce reflux.

Discospondylitis

Discospondylitis occurs when an intervertebral disc and adjacent vertebral endplates become infected. The source of infection can be from a urinary tract infection, skin infection, oral cavity infection, penetrating wounds or plant material migration – all may cause direct infection of the disc space or vertebrae.

Diagnosis

Spinal radiographs demonstrate evidence of disease, including narrowing of the disc space, with subtle irregularity of both endplates, gross lysis and osseous proliferation of the adjacent vertebral bone, and even fractures.

Clinical signs

- Spinal pain.
- Ataxia.
- Paresis.
- Systemic illness, fever and weight loss.

Treatment

- Antibiotics.
- Analgesics.
- Rest.

Physiotherapy

- Maintain joint ROM and muscle length in the limbs.
- Avoid any pressure or stress on the affected spine especially in the presence of bone changes within the vertebrae.
- Gentle standing and supported gait practice; avoid stairs and inclines as this will increase stress on the spine.

Toxoplasmosis and neosporosis

The most common cause of toxoplasmosis in dogs and cats is ingestion of infected intermediate host tissues. *Neospora* can also be contracted this way, but most animals are infected *in utero*. *Toxoplasma gondii* is an intracellular protozoan parasite of humans and other animals that can cause encephalitis in infected hosts. *Neospora caninum* is a protozoan parasite that is known to cause neurological disease in dogs.

Clinical signs

- Signs of disease are seen most frequently in young or immunocompromised animals.
- An early sign of disease may be progressive rigidity in one or more limbs as a result of myositis and neuritis.
- Ocular abnormalities may be evident.
- Neurological changes include: seizures, behavioural changes and cerebellar ataxia in infected adult dogs.

Diagnosis

Positive antibody titres in serum and the CSF.

Treatment

- 3–4 weeks of antibiotics.
- Pyrimethamine.
- Folic acid supplementation.

Physiotherapy

This will depend on the severity of the symptoms but will predominantly focus on improving function in a patient presenting with cerebellar ataxia.

- PROM exercises and stretches of the major muscle groups of the limbs to maintain joint ROM and muscle length.
- Improve stamina. This will take time in a patient with cerebellar ataxia and the exercise programme should be paced; aim for several

short sessions a day rather than one long exercise session. Keep the exercise restricted to simple walking on flat, firm, non-slip surfaces, for 5 minutes, four times daily to begin with.

- Once the patient is able to manage four short walks a day begin to introduce strengthening exercises. This may simply involve walking the patient on gentle inclines; be aware of the patient's balance as descending inclines may further challenge balance.
- Hydrotherapy using a UWT can be useful for improving strength. A member of staff should go in the treadmill with the patient to ensure the patient is safe. The patient should wear a buoyancy jacket. Begin with short-duration and slow-speed sessions. As the patient progresses the time and speed can be increased. To further strengthen the patient, add resistance using water jets.
- One of the main functions of the cerebellum is to maintain balance. If the cerebellum is affected by *Toxoplasma* or *Neospora* the patient will find balance challenging and intension tremors may be seen. The patient may even find walking through doorways and stepping up and down curbs very difficult to judge. Begin with gentle balance challenges such as stop-start walking, and changing direction.
- Limb lifting with support as necessary can be used to challenge balance and improve strength. Progress to incorporate small perturbations (nudges) towards the limb on which the patient is balancing. If possible progress to placing the limb on which the animal is balancing onto an unstable surface such as a wobble cushion, and incorporate small perturbations towards the limb the patient is balancing on. Most patients with cerebellar ataxia will not tolerate balancing on wobble boards, especially in the early stages of rehabilitation.
- Cavaletti poles can be used to encourage the patient to flex his limbs and also to think about where he is placing his limbs. Start with the poles at a low height and spaced for his normal gait stride length. As the patient progresses increase the height of the poles and reduce the space between the poles to challenge him further.

- In moving towards a discharge date and planning for the patient's home situation, begin working on functional activities such as stair climbing and getting in and out of the cars. If the patient is comfortable stepping up and down curbs progress this to a couple of steps together both up and down. Be aware that he may find balance challenging when descending stairs so keep in close to him and support him so he feels safe. As he becomes more confident increase the amount of stairs to match his home situation.
- Previously the patient may have independently jumped in and out of the car. He may not now have the strength and co-ordination for this so he will need assistance to get into and out of the car to ensure his safety. A ramp may be considered for large dogs. However, because his balance may be affected he should be allowed time to become used to the ramp, which can be steep and narrow. Start by having him walk on the ramp on a stable flat surface; once he is confident increase the incline of the ramp to a normal step height, and as his confidence grows continue to increase the height to the level of the car boot. Remember to keep in close to the patient when he is on the ramp and support him as necessary to ensure he feels safe and secure.

Physiotherapy home exercise programme for toxoplasmosis and neosporosis

Early phase (approx. 0–2 weeks)

Mobility

Controlled walking using a chest harness 5 minutes, four times daily. Allow the patient to exercise freely indoors; try avoid stairs as she will not feel safe on them due to her reduced balance.

Sitting and standing practice

Try to encourage the patient to spend some of her day sitting and standing.

Strengthening
Sit to stand exercises, two sets of 5 repetitions daily.

Balance
The patient's balance reactions may be reduced; for example, if it is the right fore limb, to improve the patient's standing balance gently nudge her at the left shoulder; her balance and strength will increase as she resists the movement.

Mid-phase (approx. 2–4 weeks)

Mobility
Start to add gentle slopes up and down and weaving between objects into the exercise plan. Five minutes, four times a day. Continue to use the chest harness and lead.

Continue with exercises from the early phase.

Late phase (4–6 weeks)

Mobility
Continue with mobility as in mid-phase; add in stepping over small logs or rolls and increase duration to 10–15 minutes four times daily. Also begin to exercise the patient on different surfaces, such as concrete, grass, bark chippings and sand. Exercising her in long grass will have a strengthening effect on the limbs as she navigates her way through it.

Continue with the exercises from mid phase.

Outpatient physiotherapy or onward referral

Outpatients would normally be seen once a week to improve stamina, strength and balance and then be re-assessed at 6 weeks.

Neurological assessment

This assessment is carried out by the veterinary surgeon, but by assisting you will gain valuable information relating to the presenting condition of the patient. The aim of the neurological assessment is to localise the lesion prior to confirming this with diagnostics. Both time and money can be saved by following a thorough neurological assessment. Requesting a full spinal MRI scan is time consuming, costly and unnecessary if the lesion can be localised to a spinal region; this region can then be the focus of the MRI diagnostics.

Subjective examination

This section includes the patient's past medical history (PMH), the history of the presenting condition (HPC), and the patient's presenting condition (PC). Most of this information will be given by the owner at the time of the initial consultation or from the referring veterinary surgeon if applicable.

Objective examination

Mentation: is the patient alert; depressed; disorientated; in a stupor; or comatose?

Posture: is this normal; head tilt to the left or right; falling to the left or right?

Gait: normal; ataxic; stiffness; dysmetria; circling to the left or right?

Limbs affected: para (two limbs); tetra (four limbs); hemi (left- or right-side limbs); or mono (one limb)?

Tone: Absent = 0; decreased = 1; normal = 2; increased = 3; clonus = 4.

Muscle bulk: compare right and left thoracic limbs; and right and left pelvic limbs.

Hip sway: towards the right pelvic limb; or the left pelvic limb?

Pain: hyperaesthesia in which region – cervical, thoracic, lumbar or lumbosacral?

Superficial pain: Assess right and left thoracic limbs; right and left pelvic limbs?

Deep pain perception: Assess right and left thoracic limbs; right and left pelvic limbs; or tail?

Spinal reflexes

Spinal reflexes test the sensory and motor components of the reflex arc. Reflexes may be decreased, which may indicate a lower motor neuron (LMN) lesion; normal; or increased, which may indicate an upper motor neuron (UMN) lesion. It is useful to grade reflexes at initial assessment to provide baseline data and to compare subsequent changes against. Generally the spinal reflex grading system is found to be most accurate if the same person carries it out each time.

Myotatic reflexes

Myotatic reflexes are local reflex arcs that do not require cerebral perception for function. The reflex arc consists of a sensory neuron that responds to a stretch of a muscle, and a motor neuron that in turn causes muscle contraction. The most common and reliable myotatic reflex is the patella (L4-L6) reflex. This is usually tested with the animal in lateral recumbency with the pelvic limb supported and slightly flexed at the stifle. The patella ligament is briskly tapped; this results in extension of the stifle. If this reflex is diminished a LMN lesion may be suspected. However, if this reflex is increased it may indicate a UMN lesion. Myotatic reflexes can also be tested at the site of the extensor carpi radialis (C7-T2), and gastrocnemius (L6-S1). However, generally these reflex sites are considered to be less reliable.

Flexor reflexes

These reflexes test limb withdrawal. The skin between the toes is pinched to stimulate the sensory neurons. The response of the sensory neurons to the stimulus may be classified as absent, normal or brisk. To assess for the presence of deep pain perception in the limb the veterinary surgeon will use a pair of haemostats on the nail bed. If deep pain perception is present the animal will react with brisk withdrawal of the test limb and may even try to turn and bite the operator. However, if deep pain is not present the animal will not react to the painful stimuli. In borderline patients it may be necessary to compare for deep pain perception in other limbs; however, because of the painful nature of this test it should only be carried out for diagnostic purposes, that is, only retest if a sudden loss of deep pain perception is suspected.

The perineal reflex may be altered with spinal lesions in the S1-S3 region. These lesions are commonly associated with road traffic accident (RTA) 'tail pull' injuries, characterised with cauda equina signs of faecal incontinence and urinary retention. Loss of anal reflex can be tested by inserting a rectal thermometer into the anus. The normal reaction is for the anus to contract when stimulated; both right and left sides should be assessed. Injuries and suspected S1-S3 lesions are emergencies requiring urgent veterinary intervention for appropriate bladder management. The bladder should be assessed for size, control and ease of expression. Voluntary tail movement and carriage should be assessed; deep pain perception can also be assessed in the tail.

The cutaneous trunci or panniculus

Testing is carried out to assess superficial spinal nerve integrity. The skin is pinched using haemostats at intervals slightly lateral to the spinal body segments to elicit a response (skin twitch). If a compressive lesion is suspected in the T3-L3 region the skin would be pinched segmentally from the level of the iliac wings moving in a cranial direction. A negative skin twitch at T11-12 would indicate a lesion at T9-10 as this reflex usually tests spinal cord segments or nerves approximately two vertebral bodies cranial to the site of the negative response (Millis et al., 2004). Both left and right sides of the vertebral column should be assessed as slight differences in skin sensation can be found with lateralised spinal compression.

Postural reactions

Postural reactions can be thought of as righting reactions, as the animal will react to a change in body position by shifting its weight to avoid falling over. A positive abnormal postural reaction may indicate a neurological disorder; however, since these reactions involve complex interactions between the brain, spinal cord and peripheral nerves, localisation of the lesion will rely on a complete neurological assessment of the patient.

Hopping

This can be used to assess postural reactions in the pelvic and thoracic limbs. This should be carried out on a non-slip floor. Hopping requires the animal to have good strength and balance in the limb that is being assessed. All four limbs should be assessed to differentiate between tetraparesis, paraparesis, hemiparesis or monoparesis of the limbs.

Wheelbarrowing

This can be carried out to assess function in the thoracic limbs by the assessor lifting and supporting the pelvic limbs and encouraging the animal to move forwards, or by lifting the thoracic limbs and encouraging the animal to move backwards. Information from this test can be used to assess strength and balance in the limbs and differentiate between tetraparesis and paraparesis.

Hemi-walking

This is carried out by lifting and supporting the animal on the lefthand side then moving the animal laterally to the righthand side to test the postural reactions of the righthand limbs. The test should also be carried out on the lefthand side for comparison and to assess a hemiparetic patient.

Conscious proprioception

This test can be carried out on all four limbs in turn to assess the animal's awareness of joint position. The animal stands squarely and is supported as necessary by the assessor. The limb to be assessed is turned over by the assessor so the animal is weight-bearing or *knuckling* on the dorsal surface of the limb. It is usual for the assessor to repeat the test three times. The normal response is for the animal to correct the paw position immediately. The response can be classified as present (normal), delayed or absent. In the thoracic limb this test would assess conscious proprioception in the carpal joint; in the pelvic limb the test would assess conscious proprioception in the tarsal joint.

A paper test can also be used to assess conscious proprioception in the proximal limb joints. The limb to be tested is placed on a thick sheet of paper, and the paper is then gently withdrawn in a caudal direction. The normal response is for the animal to step off the sheet of paper and to bring the limb forwards.

Cranial nerves (CN)

Both right and left sides should be assessed and compared (Table 2.2).

Localisation of the lesion

Findings from the neurological examination should be listed or charted to aim to localise the lesion. From this point the neurologist may request further diagnostic testing such as blood tests, electromyography (EMG) or MRI to confirm the diagnosis.

Lesions are localised as:

Central: involving the brain; they may be further localised into forebrain, brainstem, cerebellum or vestibular (which can be central or peripheral).

Table 2.2 Cranial nerve testing.

Cranial nerve	Test
2	Vision
2,3	Pupil size
2,7	Menace
3,4,6,8	Strabismus
3,4,6,8	Nystagmus
5	Facial sensory
7	Facial motor
5,7	Palpebral
9,10	Gag
12	Tongue

Spinal cord:

- C1-C5 UMN signs.
- C6-T2 LMN signs.
- T3-L3 UMN signs.
- L4-S3 normal thoraciclimbs, LMN pelvic limbs.
- L4-L5 LMN signs to femoral nerve (weak hip flexion).
- L6-S2 normal femoral nerve, LMN sciatic nerve (weak hip extension).

Peripheral

Neuromuscular

Mononeuropathy

Polyneuropathy

Junctionopathy

Myopathy

Diagnosis

Localising the lesion should provide an anatomical diagnosis and guide the choice of further investigations towards an aetiological diagnosis (Table 2.3).

Table 2.3 Grading the severity of spinal cord lesions.

Grade	Presentation of clinical signs
Grade 1	Pain only. Ambulatory with no other deficits noted
Grade 2	Tetraparesis or paraparesis. Ambulatory with loss of proprioceptive function, weakness and ataxia
Grade 3	Tetraparesis or paraparesis. Non-ambulatory, but evidence of voluntary movement in the limbs
Grade 4	Tetraparesis or paraplegia. Non-ambulatory, with no evidence of voluntary movement in the limbs, deep pain sensation present. +/– urinary function/control
Grade 5	Paraplegia. As above, with no evidence of deep pain sensation

Physiotherapy assessment for the neurology patient

The physiotherapy assessment for the neurological patient will differ from the veterinary surgeons' assessment. It is broken down into three main areas consisting of a patient database, a subjective examination and an objective examination. At the time the patient is referred for physiotherapy a diagnosis has usually been reached and given by the veterinary surgeon.

Database

History of presenting condition (HPC)

Typical questions to ask the owner in this section may include:

- Was the animal involved in any traumatic incident prior to the onset of symptoms?
- Did the symptoms develop over a period of time? Or is this an acute presentation?
- Is the animal improving, deteriorating or are the symptoms staying the same?

Past medical injury (PMH)

Typical questions to ask the owner in this section may include:

- Has the animal had this condition or similar symptoms before?
- Does the animal have any other concurrent disease? (Animals with bilateral cruciate disease may present with pelvic limb weakness and reduced conscious proprioception, meaning that they may appear to present neurologically, when in fact this would be an orthopaedic presentation.)

Drug history (DH)

This section is important if the patient has been on long-term medications such as steroids or anti-epileptic drugs. Ask if the patient is currently on any analgesics, and if so are these making a difference?

Results of specific investigations

- Radiographs.
- CT scans.
- MRI.
- Blood tests.

This information will usually be found in the patient's file.

Subjective examination

Explore the owner's ability to manage the patient once the patient is discharged.

- Assess the patient's home situation (access to garden, stairs in the house, other animals in the house, ability to get in and out of car if necessary).
- What was his daily exercise regime? Explain that this will probably need to be adapted and several short walks per day may be preferable to one long walk per day.
- Is the animal in pain? Pain scoring scales such as the Glasgow Composite Measure Pain Scale Short Form (GCMPS-SF) can be used to measure pain in dogs.

- What are the owner's main concerns for the patient? This may be how the owner will manage the dog in and out of the car.
- What are the owner's expectations of physiotherapy? Do they expect a 100% recovery for their pet, or do they expect to make changes and adaptions for their pet?

The subjective examination is an important section that can be overlooked or not taken into consideration. For example, a miniature dachshund undergoing spinal surgery will have different needs to a great Dane undergoing spinal surgery. Issues such as stairs and getting out to the garden may not be problematic for small dogs as the owners will be able to carry the dog up the stairs and out to the garden. However, consideration should be given to how a giant dog recovering from spinal surgery will be managed by the owner in the home situation.

Objective examination

Posture

This will take into account spinal alignment; is the patient's posture normal or is scoliosis, kyphosis or lordosis present? How does the patient distribute his weight in stance; is he shifting weight from weak limbs?

Sitting balance

Does the animal have independent sitting balance? Does he sit in a normal position with his pelvic limbs flexed under his pelvis? Or with the pelvic limbs flexed at the hips with stifle extension and a flexed thoracolumbar spine, typically seen with spinal patients?

Standing balance

Does the animal have independent standing balance or does he need assistance? Is he weak in all limbs, or only his pelvic limbs (tetraparesis vs paraparesis).

Hopping ability

This test is used to assess balance, strength and control of the limbs. Hopping ability is often impaired in neurological patients.

Voluntary movements

Assess the strength of voluntary movements, and the stamina of the patient. If he is paretic he will tire easily and may have a crouched gait pattern. Is he ataxic in his pelvic limbs, or hypermetric in his thoracic limbs?

Involuntary movements

Tremor may be present if the cerebellum is affected. This may be observed when the animal is sitting or standing still; slight involuntary movements of the head may be observed. Involuntary movements are often seen in epileptic or seizuring patients.

Tone

Increased: this may be associated with upper motor neuron lesions (spinal segments C1-C5 and T3-L3).

Decreased: this may be associated with lower motor neuron lesions (spinal segments C6-T2 and L4-S3).

Spasticity: presents as abnormally high tone that is difficult break down with PROM exercises. It can be associated with muscle weakness when the animal increases his muscle tone to assist him to stand and mobilise (when working against gravity). In these cases muscle tone should be found to be normal when in a gravity eliminated position (i.e. lying down).

Rigidity: this may be seen as flexor or extensor rigidity, as observed in brain injury and tetanus patients. Abnormal prolonged muscle activity will lead to contractions, and abnormal changes in the associated joints.

Reflexes

Flexor reflexes: thoracic C6-T2, pelvic L6-S2 (withdrawal).

Myotatic reflexes: extensor carpi radialis C7-T2, patella L4-L6, gastrocnemius L6–S1, perineal S1-S3.

Reflexes may be graded as: 0 = absent, 1 = weak, 2 = normal, 3 = brisk, and 4 = clonus.

Muscle length and joint range

Passive joint ROM can be measured with a goniometer. If muscles become short and tight this can reduce the ROM of the joint(s) associated with that muscle; for example, short hip flexors will lead to reduced hip extension.

Muscle bulk

Muscle bulk is measured around the circumference of the muscle belly using a standard tape measure. When measuring muscle bulk, for example the left pelvic limb, always also measure the muscle bulk in the right pelvic limb to compare differences, and for evaluating subsequent outcome measure changes.

Sensory awareness

Light touch: does the patient respond to gentle touch? Is this consistent throughout the limb or is it most obvious, for example, on the medial surface of the thoracic limb when compared to the lateral surface? Dermatome patterns are associated with specific nerves, so if nerve root C8, which innervates the lateral aspect of the thoracic limb, is compromised the patient may have altered sensation in this region.

Temperature: if the patient has altered sensation be aware that this may affect his ability to notice changes in temperature in the affected region. This can be very important if hot or cold packs are being applied to the affected area for any reason.

Conscious proprioception

See earlier notes on veterinary surgeon neurological patient assessment under 'Neurological assessment'.

Panniculus cut-off or cutaneous trunci

This is a test to assess sensation of dermatomes within the thoracolumbar region of the spinal column. Haemostats are used to pinch the skin along the side of the spinal column, starting caudally at the level of the wings of the ilium and moving cranially segmentally; both sides of the spinal column are assessed in turn to localise the site of the lesion. The normal reaction would be for the patient to twitch the area of skin being pinched by the haemostats. Areas of skin caudal to the lesion will not react to the stimuli, or may show a weak response. Areas cranial to the lesion should demonstrate a definite skin twitch. The junction between stimulus reaction and stimulus non-reaction would indicate a lesion two vertebral spaces cranial to the junction. The lesion may be on the left or right of the spinal column, so both left and right sides should be assessed.

Functional activities

- Assess the patient's ability to independently change position and turn onto left and right sides.
- Does the patient have independent sitting and standing balance?
- Is the patient able to lie, sit, stand and walk independently?
- Assess the patient's ability to ascend/descend stairs, if appropriate.
- Assess the patient's ability to jump in/out of a car, if appropriate.

Is the patient independent in these activities or can he complete them with assistance from someone else?

Gait

- Is the patient ambulatory or non-ambulatory? (Ambulatory means he mobilises without assistance from anyone or without the use of the aid of slings, etc.)
- If the patient is non-ambulatory, can he mobilise with the use of slings/walking aids and assistance from others? If he needs assistance note if this is maximum, moderate or minimum.

Other features

Pattern: is the patient ataxic or hypermetric?
Distance: how far can the patient mobilise; is he paretic (weak)?

Exercise tolerance/fatigue: does the patient have decreased stamina? Does he sit and rest after a short distance?

Mental status: is the patient mentally alert? Is his behaviour appropriate or inappropriate to the situation?

Self-assessment questions

1 PROM exercises are predominantly performed to:
  - **a** Maintain strength in the affected limbs.
  - **b** Maintain joint ROM in the affected limbs.
  - **c** Improve (lengthen) muscle.
  - **d** Improve blood flow to the affected limbs.

2 Stretching muscles aims to:
  - **a** Maintain or increase muscle length.
  - **b** Improve blood flow to the area.
  - **c** Improve muscle strength.
  - **d** Reduce blood flow to the area.

3 In which of the following situations might hydrotherapy be contraindicated?
  - **a** The patient underwent a hemi-laminectomy (HLE) 9 days ago; the surgical site has healed but skin staples are still present at the surgical site.
  - **b** The patient has a grade II heart murmur (no clinical signs are present and he is not on any medication for this).
  - **c** The patient currently has a urinary tract infection.
  - **d** The patient does not like deep water

4 Tetraparesis is a term used to describe:
  - **a** Weakness in one limb.
  - **b** Weakness in the limbs on the left or right side of the body.
  - **c** Weakness in the pelvic limbs.
  - **d** Weakness in all four limbs.

5 Where would you localise a lesion to in a tetraparetic patient?
  - **a** C1-C5
  - **b** T3-L3

c L4-S1
d S1-S3

6 Which cranial nerves control pupil size and can be stimulated by light?
a 2, 3
b 5, 7
c 6, 8
d 9, 10

7 Myasthenia gravis is classified as a:
a Neuromuscular disease
b Cerebellar disease
c Forebrain disease
d Brainstem disease

8 How would a fibrocartilaginous embolism (FCE) be classified?
a Degenerative
b Neoplastic
c Idiopathic
d Vascular

9 Which exercise would best challenge/improve proprioception?
a Wobble board
b Cavaletti poles
c Stairs
d Weaving cones

10 Which position should a patient be in when assessing muscle tone?
a Supported over a peanut-type physio ball.
b Supported by a hoist in an underwater treadmill.
c A side lying position.
d Supported by two people using slings to maintain the patient in a standing position.

CHAPTER 3

Respiratory physiotherapy

Introduction

Respiratory physiotherapy is probably the least recognised and least understood treatment used in veterinary patients. The aims of treatment are to:

- Clear chest secretions
- Improve gaseous exchange
- Increase lung volume
- Reduce respiratory effort
- Improve exercise tolerance
- Prevent secondary complications.

These aims are achieved by using manual techniques such as percussion (coupage) and vibrations to clear secretions, and positioning to optimise gaseous exchange and prevent secondary respiratory complications.

Practical Physiotherapy for Veterinary Nurses, First Edition. Donna Carver.

Chest auscultation and interpretation

Chest auscultation should be carried out in a quiet area. Ideally the patient is positioned either standing or sitting; if this is not possible then he may rest in sternal recumbency. It is preferable if the patient is not panting; however, be aware that the patient may be panting because he is in respiratory distress, and closing his mouth to auscultate his chest may cause him further distress.

A systematic approach should be adopted comparing left and right sides. Dogs and cats have four lung lobes on the right side, and three lung lobes on the left side. It is not always possible to be sure which lung lobe you are auscultating over, so it is easier to divide the lung fields into zones. Each lung should be divided into three zones: the upper zone is the area of lung cranial to the heart, the mid-zone the area of lung over the heart, and the lower zone the area of lung tissue caudal to the heart.

Breath sounds

Normal breath sounds tend to be quiet, with a inspiration / expiration ratio of 1:2; inspiration is the shorter, followed without a pause by a longer expiration phase, which tends to be passive.

Diminished sounds or quiet breath sounds may be evident in areas of atelectasis caused by reduced air entry into the affected area. Diminished breath sounds may also be evident over pleural effusions, as the fluid within the pleural space will *muffle* the normal sounds, or if pneumothorax is present and gaseous exchange is compromised.

Added sounds

Fine crackles may be evident when auscultating towards the lower zones (or bases) of the lungs and towards the periphery of the lung zones. A fine, sharp crack may be heard at the end of inspiration just before expiration, and is caused by a small amount of fluid in the alveoli and peripheral airways when pulmonary oedema is present.

Coarse crackles are associated with retention of secretions in the larger proximal airways. Early inspiratory and expiratory coarse crackles are evident in bronchitis; late inspiratory coarse crackles are evident with pneumonia.

It is worth remembering that the worse or louder the respiratory noise is in patients with pneumonia the easier it will be to clear the secretions using manual techniques. If the secretions are not cleared and the area of lung tissue becomes consolidated, air entry and lung volume will be reduced. This will result in an increase in respiratory rate and a drop in pulse oximetry oxygen saturation (SPO_2) values, and secretion clearance using manual techniques will be more difficult.

Wheeze is evident with narrowing of the airways; an expiratory wheeze with prolonged expiration is often associated with asthma. A wheeze during both inspiration and expiration may indicate an airway stricture.

Many educational websites are available with audible auscultation breath sounds, including the Colorado State University Auscultation Library (http://www.cvmbs.colostate.edu/clinsci/callan/breath_sounds.htm).

Percussion note technique and interpretation

The percussion note is tested to determine if air, fluid or solid structures are present within the lungs. The operator places a middle finger between the patients rib space and sharply taps the distal end of his finger with the other hand. The percussion note may be:

- *Resonant* and therefore normal.
- *Hyperresonant*, which may indicate emphysema or pneumothorax.
- *Dull*, indicating areas of consolidation, collapse or pleural effusion.

The percussion note test is usually performed along with other diagnostic tests and is not a reliable diagnostic tool when used alone.

Interpretation of blood gases

Acidosis

Acidosis is an increase in blood acidity, and blood pH is determined by the blood acid–alkali balance. The P_aCO_2 is the measure of partial pressure of carbon dioxide in arterial blood; an increase of P_aCO_2 indicates respiratory acidosis; a decreased level of HCO_3 (bicarbonate) in blood indicates a metabolic acidosis.

Alkalosis

Alkalosis occurs when the blood pH increases. A decrease in P_aCO_2 indicates a respiratory alkalosis. An increase in HCO_3 indicates a metabolic alkalosis.

Base excess

Base excess assesses the metabolic component of acid–base disturbances and indicates the degree of renal compensation. A reduced base excess indicates a metabolic acidosis and an increase in base excess indicates a metabolic alkalosis (Kenyon & Kenyon, 2009) (Table 3.1).

The blood pH will be altered in uncompensated acid–base disorders, whereas pH will be normal in compensated acid–base disorders (Table 3.2).

Respiratory failure

Respiratory failure occurs when blood gas values cannot be maintained within normal limits (Table 3.3). There are two types.

Type I (hypoxaemic respiratory failure)

This is characterised by a decrease in the partial pressure of oxygen in arterial blood (P_aO_2: hypoxaemia) with a normal or slightly increased P_aCO_2 due to inadequate gas exchange. Causes include:

- Pneumonia
- Emphysema
- Severe asthma.

Table 3.1 Normal blood values.

Parameter	Reference range canine	Reference range feline
Arterial blood analysis		
pH	7.395 [±0.03]	7.34 [±0.1]
P_aO_2 (mmHg)	102.1 [±6.8]	102.9 [±15]
P_aCO_2 (mmHg)	36.8 [±2.7]	33.6 [±7]
HCO_3 (mmol/L)	21.4 [±1.6]	17.5 [±3]
Base excess (mmol/L)	−1.8 [±1.6]	−6.4 [±5]
Venous blood analysis		
pH	7.352 [±0.02]	7.30 [±0.08]
P_aO_2 (mmHg)	55 [±9.6]	36.8 [±11]
P_aCO_2 (mmHg)	42.1 [±4.4]	41.8 [±9]
HCO_3 (mmol/L)	22.1 [±2]	19.4 [±4]
Base excess (mmol/L)	−2.1 [±1.7]	−5.7 [±5]

Adapted from Waddell, L.S. (2013) The practitioner's acid–base primer: obtaining & interpreting blood gases. *Today's Veterinary Practice*, May/June. Reprinted with permission of the North American Veterinary Community.

Table 3.2 Simple acid–base disorders.

	pH	P_aCO_2	HCO_3
Respiratory acidosis			
Uncompensated	Decreased	Increased	Normal
Compensated	Normal	Increased	Increased
Respiratory alkalosis			
Uncompensated	Increased	Decreased	Normal
Compensated	Normal	Decreased	Decreased
Metabolic acidosis			
Uncompensated	Decreased	Normal	Decreased
Compensated	Normal	Decreased	Decreased
Metabolic alkalosis			
Uncompensated	Increased	Normal	Increased
Compensated	Normal	Increased	Increased

Table 3.3 Arterial blood gas classification of respiratory failure.

	pH	P_aCO_2	HCO_3
Acute	Decreased	Increased	Normal
Chronic	Normal	Increased	Increased
Acute on chronic	Decreased	Increased	Increased

Acute or chronic relates to either type I or II respiratory failure. Acute on chronic would occur in a patient who has either chronic type I or II respiratory failure that is generally managed well medically but has an exacerbation of symptoms; e.g. when a patient with chronic emphysema is taken for a long run the chronic emphysema may become exacerbated, in which case it is termed acute on chronic.

Type II (ventilatory failure)

This is characterised by a decreased P_aO_2 with an increased P_aCO_2 (hypercapnia) caused by hypoventilation. Causes include:

- Polyradiculoneuritis.
- Asthma, chronic obstructive pulmonary disease (COPD).
- Drug-related respiratory drive depression (Kenyon & Kenyon, 2009).

Cardiorespiratory monitoring

Cardiorespiratory monitoring and recording shows trends over time. Observing the trends over a period of time allows for early intervention to forestall a crisis situation.

Arterial blood pressure (ABP) is measured via an intra-arterial cannula for continuous monitoring; the cannula also provides access for arterial blood sampling for blood gas analysis.

Cardiac output (CO) is the volume of blood pumped into the aorta each minute (Table 3.4).

Central venous pressure (CVP) measures circulating blood volume and venous return via a cannula placed in the jugular vein.

Table 3.4 Cardiorespiratory monitoring equations.

Parameter	Equation
Cardiac output (CO) (L/min)	CO = HR × SV
Cerebral perfusion pressure (CPP) (mmHg)	CPP = MAP– ICP
Mean arterial pressure (MAP) (mmHg)	MAP = (diastolic BP × 2) + (systolic BP)/3
Stroke volume (SV) (mL)	SV = (CO × 1000)/HR
Systemic vascular resistance (SVR) (mmHg)	SVR = (MAP – CVP/CO) × 79.9

BP, blood pressure (mmHg); CVP, central venous pressure (mmHg); ICP, intracranial pressure (mmHg).

Cerebral perfusion pressure (CPP) is used to measure blood supply to the brain.

Heart rate (HR) is defined as the number of times the heart beats per minute.

Intracranial pressure (ICP) is the pressure exerted on the brain by the cerebrospinal fluid (CSF). Hydrocephalus, cerebral haemorrhage, hypoxia and infection cause the ICP to rise resulting in a decreased blood supply to the brain. The patient may show signs of altered mentation; handling of the patient should be kept to a minimum, and ideally the head should be supported at a 15–30° angle to prevent further ICP.

Mean arterial pressure (MAP) is the average measure of blood in the circulatory system, related to cardiac output and systemic vascular resistance. MAP is an indicator of the tissue perfusion pressure.

Oxygen saturation (SPO_2) is the measure of arterial blood oxygen saturation expressed as a percentage using non-invasive pulse oximetry.

Respiratory rate (RR) is a measure of the number of breaths in 1 minute.

Stroke volume (SV) relates to the volume of blood ejected from the ventricles during each systolic contraction.

Systemic vascular resistance (SVR) measures vascular overload in the left ventricle. Vasoconstriction will increase systemic vascular resistance, vasodilation will decrease it.

Electrocardiograms

Electrocardiograms (ECGs) detect the sequence of electrical events that occur during the contraction (depolarisation) and relaxation (repolarisation) cycle of the heart. Depolarisation is initiated by the sinoatrial node, the heart's natural pacemaker, which transmits the electrical stimulus to the atrioventricular (AV) node. From here the impulse is conducted through the bundle of His and along the bundle branches to the Purkinje fibres, causing the heart to contract.

Normal sinus rhythm is characterised by:

- Regular rhythms and rates.
- A P wave, QRS complex and T wave are all present; and all similar in size and shape (Figure 3.1).

Sinus tachycardia (Figure 3.2) occurs with sinus rhythm and an elevated resting heart. Causes include:

- Sepsis
- Anaemia
- Pulmonary embolism

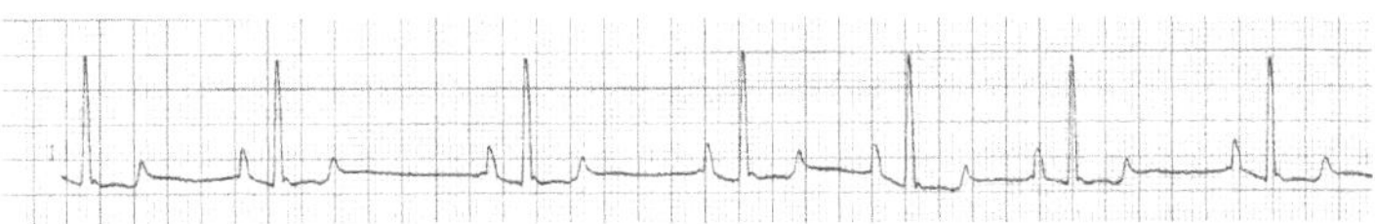

Figure 3.1 Electrocardiogram of normal sinus rhythm.

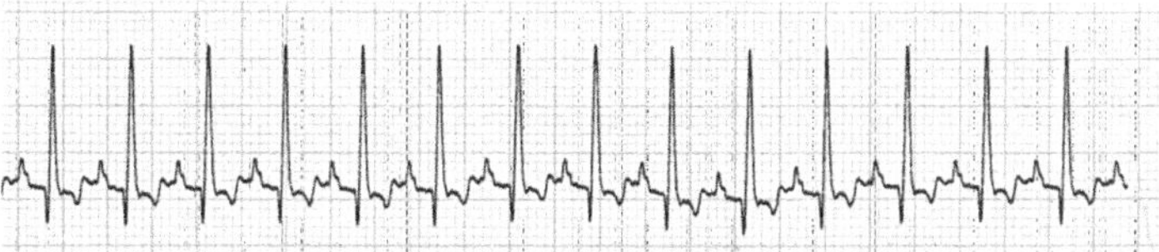

Figure 3.2 Electrocardiogram of sinus tachycardia.

- Hypovolaemia
- Drugs (salbutamol).

Sinus tachycardia can also occur in high emotional states such as:

- Pain
- Anxiety
- Fear.

Premature ventricular contractions (PVCs) are characterised by early beats (ectopic), usually caused by electrical irritability in the ventricular conduction system or myocardium. They can be asymptomatic. However, they can indicate impending fatal arrhythmias in patients with heart disease. ECG findings include:

- An irregular rhythm during PVC; however, underlying rhythm and rate are usually regular.
- The P wave is absent, the QRS complex is wide and early, and the T wave is in the opposite direction from the QRS complex during PVC (Figure 3.3).

Atrial fibrillation is characterised by rapid unsynchronised electrical activity generated in the atrial tissue. Transmission of the impulses to the ventricles via the AV node is variable and unpredictable, leading to an irregular heartbeat. ECG findings include:

- Absent P waves replaced by fine baseline oscillations.
- Irregular ventricular complexes.
- Ventricular rate varies between 100 and 180 bpm but can be slower (Figure 3.4).

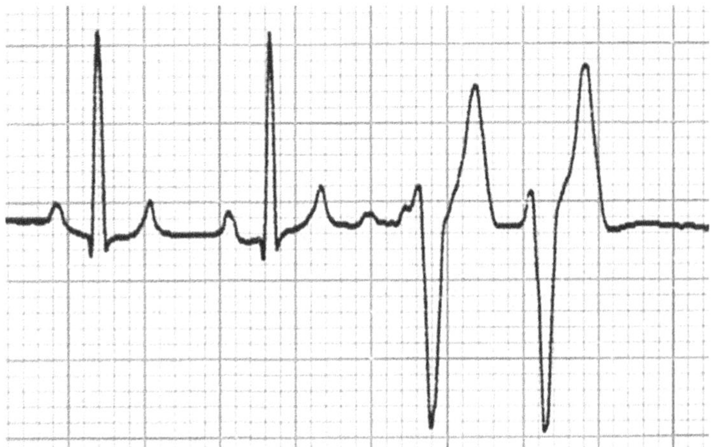

Figure 3.3 Electrocardiogram of premature ventricular contractions.

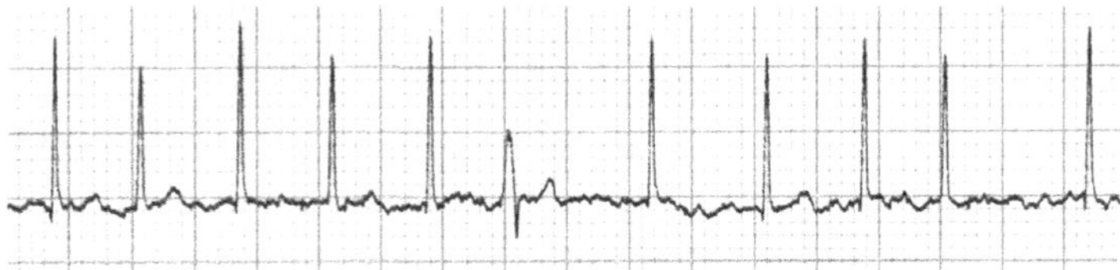

Figure 3.4 Electrocardiogram of atrial fibrillation.

Respiratory presenting conditions

Chronic obstructive pulmonary disease (COPD)

Chronic obstructive pulmonary disease (COPD) is an umbrella term used to describe several relatively common respiratory diseases affecting humans, in which it is often associated with tobacco smoking or contact with fine particles that may be inhaled into the lungs, such as asbestos. Domestic animals may be subjected to passive smoking, which may contribute to COPD in these species (Figure 3.5).

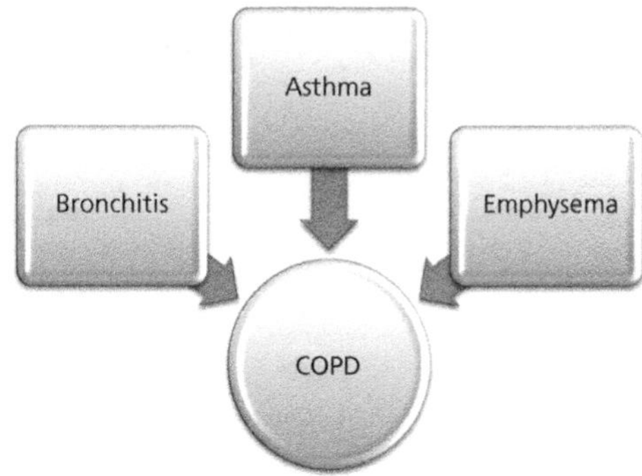

Figure 3.5 Chronic obstructive pulmonary disease.

Asthma

Asthma tends to be seen more commonly in feline patients. Diagnosis is usually reached by eliminating other diseases and by the response seen to treatment (anti-inflammatory steroids). Symptoms include increased respiratory rate and effort in the expiratory phase as the patient attempts to clear CO_2 from the lungs. Nebulisation is not usually indicated and may even exacerbate the symptoms. The patients do not usually struggle with oxygenation, but have difficulty with expiration to clear CO_2, and the pressure from the fine flow of moist particles produced by the nebuliser will make expiration more difficult for these patients.

Bronchitis

Bronchitis is inflammation of the bronchi. This inflammatory process may result in excessive secretions being produced. If the animal is unable to cough and clear these secretions he may show signs of respiratory compromise, seen as an increase in respiratory rate and effort, especially apparent on expiration. Arterial blood gases may be altered and the patient may develop a respiratory acidosis. On

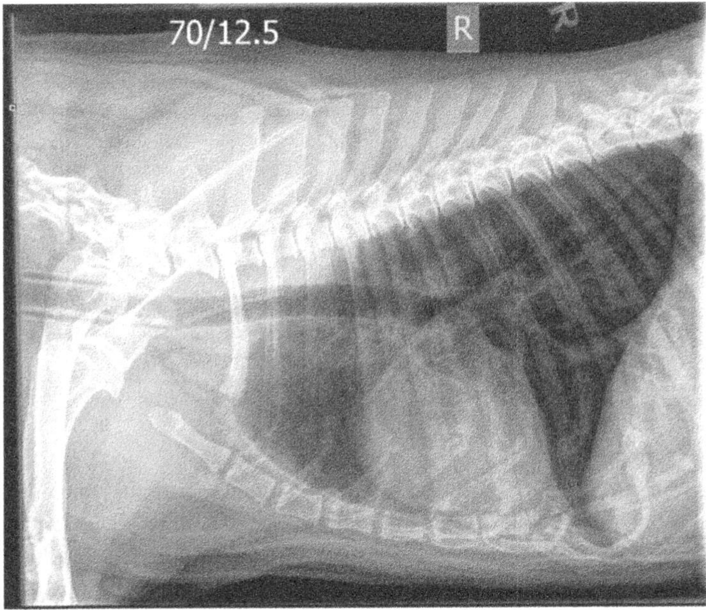

Figure 3.6 X-ray of bronchitis showing a moderate diffuse bronchial pattern.

auscultation *coarse crackles* will be evident over the large airways, with an extended expiratory phase (Figure 3.6).

Emphysema

Emphysema is seen in patients with COPD. They often have a *barrel-shaped chest*, which develops over time as the patient acquires a very large lung volume; unfortunately this increased lung volume is not all functional or compliant with respiratory gas exchange. The patient will show increased respiratory rate with an increased expiratory phase in an attempt to blow off CO_2. The patient may have altered arterial blood gases and show a respiratory acidosis. SPO_2 is usually decreased; however, care should be taken when these patients are supplemented with oxygen as their high blood CO_2 levels act as a respiratory drive, and it may be *normal* for them to have a low SPO_2 of around 95%. If these patients are over-supplemented with oxygen they may lose their respiratory drive function.

Pneumonia

Pneumonia is seen relatively commonly in animals (Figure 3.7). It may be a *bacterial pneumonia* if the animal develops an infection. Symptoms include pyrexia, loss of appetite and lethargy; a moist, often productive cough may be present.

Hypostatic pneumonia is often associated with recumbent animals, who may lie on one side for a long period of time resulting in the dependent lung becoming compressed and resulting in a loss of functional lung volume in this lung. Patients often show an increase in respiratory rate, a reduced SPO_2, reduced chest expansion and altered arterial blood gases.

Aspiration pneumonia occurs when the patient inhales fluid into the lungs. This may be seen in patients with mega-oesophagus, who have a delayed swallow and associated reflux. Symptoms may include pyrexia, loss of appetite, increased respiratory rate,decreased SPO_2, and added sounds or *crackles* evident on auscultation.

Do not allow patients with pneumonia to become dehydrated. If the patient becomes dehydrated the chest secretions will become viscous and more difficult to clear from the chest using physiotherapy manual techniques. Nebulising patients using saline prior to treatment may be beneficial in loosening secretions, and prevent the affected lung lobes from becoming consolidated.

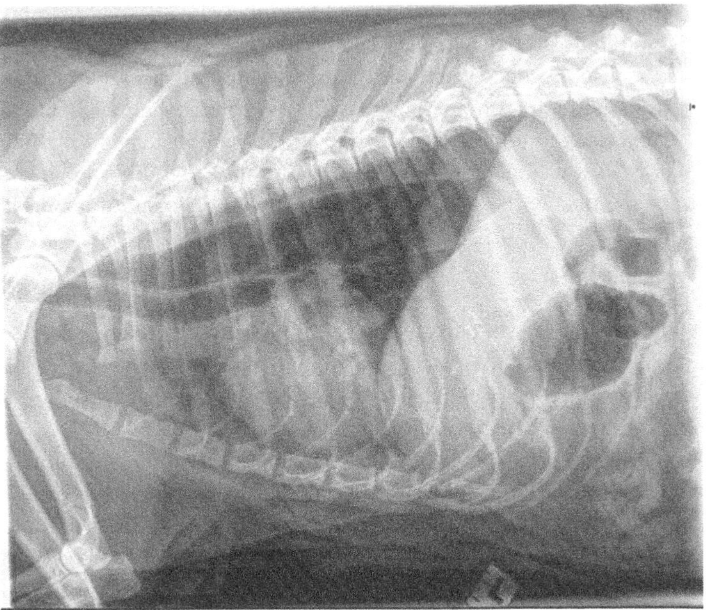

Figure 3.7 X-ray showing increased opacity over the ventral thorax with areas of alveolar pattern suggestive of pneumonia.

Respiratory physiotherapy treatment techniques

Percussion (coupage)

Percussion is a manual technique used to aid clearance of chest secretions in patients (see Appendix 2). It is only necessary to perform percussion over the affected area as indicated by chest auscultation and by reviewing chest radiographs. The patient should be positioned in sternal recumbency, sitting or standing (it is more difficult for a patient to cough and clear secretions if he is lying in lateral recumbency). If the patient has been in the same position for a period of time it may be beneficial to mobilise him for a short distance to loosen any secretions; this gentle mobility alone may be sufficient to stimulate a cough and encourage the patient to take deeper breaths to increase his lung volume and improve his oxygenation. If the patient is unable to stand and mobilise, assist him into sitting several times to attempt to loosen the secretions prior to performing percussion. If the patient is very thin (such as a whippet) place a towel over the chest to prevent any bruising to the skin; using a vetbed™ during percussion would provide too much padding so avoid this.

Use a cupped hand as this is more effective than a flat hand. Begin by applying percussion to the affected area, gently to begin with so as not to alarm the patient, then gradually increase the force. Remember the goal is to stimulate the patient to cough and clear secretions, so if you are too gentle the treatment will not be effective. Aim to apply each percussion repetition at approximately 1-second intervals; any faster than this and the patient will not have the opportunity to cough and clear secretions. It is not necessary or effective to use a caudal to cranial or bilateral technique. When the patient coughs to clear secretions it will not happen in stages or by peristalsis. Bilateral techniques are not indicated if auscultation and radiographs only demonstrate one unilateral lung lobe to be affected.

Vibrations

Vibrations are often used in conjunction with and often following percussion. The aim is to shear secretions from the airways. Vibrations can be effective when treating patients with bronchitis as the secretions may be adhered to the bronchi. The patient should be in sternal recumbency. Each of the operator's hands are placed flat on either side of the patient's chest to ensure maximum surface area is covered;

do not grip the patient. The vibrations are generated from the pectoral muscles of the operator and transmitted down the arms; they last for 2–3 seconds and are repeated for up to 1 minute. When the technique is carried out correctly the patient may appear to be trembling during the vibration treatment. Following vibration treatment encourage the patient to mobilise, to further loosen the secretions and cough to clear them.

Shaking

Shaking is similar to vibrations but uses a larger amplitude of movement. It is recommended that only a physiotherapist carries out this treatment so as not to cause injury to the patient. Again the aim is to loosen chest secretions, and encouraging the patient to cough.

Breathing exercises

Many humans with COPD are taught breathing exercises. However, it is difficult to teach animals breathing techniques. Animals will usually adapt to situations well and given the right environment they will often find the best position for maximum effective gaseous exchange. Encourage animals to change their position frequently to prevent hypostatic pneumonia. Mobilise the patient regularly to encourage secretion clearage; mobilising the patient will also encourage him to take deeper breaths, and therefore maintain his lung volume.

Assisted cough

This is also a technique used in human patients, often in patients with neurological conditions and muscular weakness who may have, or be at risk of pneumonia. The idea is to encourage the patient to take a deep breath in, and then the operator applies upward pressure under the ribs to the diaphragm as the patient is asked to quickly breathe out again. This passive upward thrust on the weak patient diaphragm may stimulate a cough and encourage the patient to clear secretions.

Positioning

Correct positioning of the patient can maximise lung volume, lung compliance and the ventilation/perfusion (V/Q) ratio. It can also reduce the patient's respiratory effort, and aid secretion clearance and coughing (Kenyon & Kenyon, 2009).

Correct positioning of a patient can be very beneficial especially when manual techniques such as percussion or vibrations are contraindicated, for example in cases of chest trauma or recent thoracic surgery.

When positioning a patient the dependent lung (the side the patient is lying on) will be better perfused; the non-dependent or uppermost lung will be better ventilated. So, if a patient has pneumonia affecting the right mid-zone he would benefit from being positioned on his left side, so the left lung would be better perfused, whilst the right lung would be better ventilated. If both sides of the chest are affected the patient should be placed in sternal recumbency.

N.B. Animals with respiratory comprise should not be placed in a ventrodorsal position, for example to obtain a "quick chest x-ray" as this will further reduce the compromised lung's ventilation capacity, by perfusing rather than ventilating the large dorsal lung fields.

Respiratory physiotherapy assessment

Database

History of presenting condition (HPC): Did the patient suddenly become ill, or was the onset of symptoms gradual but progressive?

Past medical history (PMH): Does the patient have any known cardiorespiratory conditions?

Drug history (DH): Is the patient currently on any medication (e.g. diuretics)?

Social history (SH): Are there any other dogs in the household? Is the dog left alone for periods of time while the owner is at work; what is the patient's normal exercise regime?

Subjective assessment

Main concerns: The owner may be concerned about exercise tolerance, or if the patient is exhibiting polyuria/polydipsia (PUPD) and needs to go outside frequently.

Symptoms: Coughing, inappetence, shortness of breath.

Exercise tolerance: Is it increased, the same or decreased? Is the pace fast or slow? Is the distance walked long or short before fatigue occurs?

Position: Note if the patient is standing, sitting or lying? Is he in sternal or lateral recumbency?

Lines and drains: Be aware of the position of any ECG leads, intravenous lines and chest drains.

Ability to vocalise: Is the dog able to bark, has the bark changed (become weaker), or is he unable to vocalise?

Presence of wheeze/cough: Is the wheeze on inspiration and expiration? Is the cough dry and non-productive or moist and productive?

Sputum:

Volume: Indicate volume +, ++, +++.

Consistency: Gives an indication of hydration status, and relates to ease of clearance.

Colour: Clear = saliva. Mucoid = white (chronic bronchitis without infection). Mucopurulent = slightly discoloured (pneumonia). Purulent = yellow/green/brown/rust (*Pseudomonas, Mycoplasma*). Frothy = pink or white (pulmonary oedema). Haemoptysis = blood steaks to frank blood (infection, bronchiectasis, vasculitis, cardiac disease). Black specks = smoke inhalation (coal dust).

Chest shape, breathing pattern and effort: Is the chest barrel-shaped (to increase lung volume, i.e. in emphysema)?

Objective assessment

Review chest X-rays (CXRs) and other diagnostic images: remember that the CXR can have a 24-hour time lag either way so be guided by the full clinical signs.

Heart rate (HR): Is it normal, tachycardia or bradycardia?

Temperature: Is it normal, pyrexia, hypothermic?

Respiration rate (RR): Is it normal, bradypnoea, tachypnoea?

Mucous membrane colour and capillary refill time (CRT): Pale pink, dark pink, brick red; CRT of <2 seconds is considered normal.

Oxygen therapy/humidification: Note volume of O_2 supplementation; mode (e.g. nasal prongs) and the time started on O_2; and response to therapy. Is the patient improving, remaining static or becoming worse?

SPO_2: Measured as a percentage. Note if the patient is on O_2 therapy and the volume of O_2 in L/min. If the patient has an SPO_2 around 90% on 4 L/min O_2 be concerned; remember that the SPO_2 could be considerably less were the patient not on O_2 therapy.

Blood pressure (BP): The readings will be most accurate if the patient is not stressed at the time of measurement. Ensure the cuff size and limb used are also recorded in the notes for consistency. Usually systolic, diastolic and the mean arterial pressure are measured. It is usual to discard the first reading, then take a series of five readings, and record the average BP measured from these readings.

Bodyweight: The patient should be weighed daily and the weight should be recorded in his notes. Any significant weight loss or gain should be highlighted and further investigated.

Fluid balance: Note any intravenous fluid therapy the patient is receiving and the rate of fluid therapy. His oral fluid intake should also be measured and recorded. His daily maintenance fluid requirements, plus any fluid losses (in cases of vomiting or diarrhoea) should be recorded to ensure he is not becoming dehydrated.

Urine output: Can be measured accurately if the patient has an indwelling urinary catheter attached to a collection system, otherwise urine output can be estimated.

Medications: Note any relevant medication the patient is on and the times he receives his medication.

High dependency unit (HDU)/intensive care unit (ICU) charts

Heart rhythm: Does the patient have a normal heart rhythm, or a dysrhythmia?

Inspiration:expiration (I:E) ratio: Is normally 1:2. This may change to 1:1 if the patient is hyperventilating, or to 1:3 if the patient is hypercapnic.

Oedema: Does the patient have peripheral oedema? Is he being over infused?

Chest expansion: Is this equal on the left and right sides? Note that in cases of unilateral pneumothorax the affected side will be hyperinflated with maximum chest expansion but little respiratory movement. If areas of lung are consolidated with a loss of lung volume chest expansion will be reduced

Percussion note: Record as dull (areas of consolidation), resonant (normal) or hyperresonant (pneumothorax).

Auscultation: Compare both sides for normal breath sounds throughout. Record any areas of added sounds (i.e. crackles) or diminished sounds (i.e. consolidation).

Glasgow Coma Scale (GCS): Is a 3–15-point scale used to measure the patient's level of consciousness. A total score of 3 would indicate no response to stimulus, a total score or 15 would indicate a high level of response to stimulus (See appendix 1).

Arterial blood gases (ABGs): Serial samples will show the patient's blood gas trends over time.

Blood chemistry: Results will indicate the patient's renal and hepatic function.

Chest X-rays

Pneumothorax occurs when air enters the pleural space caused by a lesion in the lung or trauma to the chest, which causes the lung to collapse. Clinical signs include acute pain, dyspnoea and decreased chest expansion on the affected side. Pneumothorax is classified by cause; three types are recognised (Kenyon & Kenyon, 2009):

- *Spontaneous pneumothorax:* Caused by rupture of the emphysematous bulla, in association with asthma, pneumonia or COPD.
- *Traumatic pneumothorax:* Caused by traumatic injury to the chest, e.g. perforation of lung tissue by fractured ribs.
- *Tension pneumothorax:* Occurs when pressure within the pleural cavity increases as a result of a tear in the visceral pleura acting as a one-way valve, allowing air to enter on inspiration but preventing it from escaping on expiration. Clinical signs include increased respiratory distress, cyanosis, hypotension and tachycardia.

Pleural effusion occurs when fluid accumulates within the pleural cavity (Figure 3.8); causes include:

- Increased hydrostatic pressure, e.g. congestive heart failure.
- Increased capillary permeability, e.g. inflammation of the pleura.
- Decreased plasma oncotic pressure, e.g. malnutrition.
- Impaired lymphatic absorption, e.g. malignancy.
- Communication with peritoneal space and fluid, e.g. ascites.

The fluid may be clear/straw-coloured *transudate* with a low protein content, indicating a disturbance of the normal pressure within the lung. Or it may be cloudy in colour and known as *exudate* with a

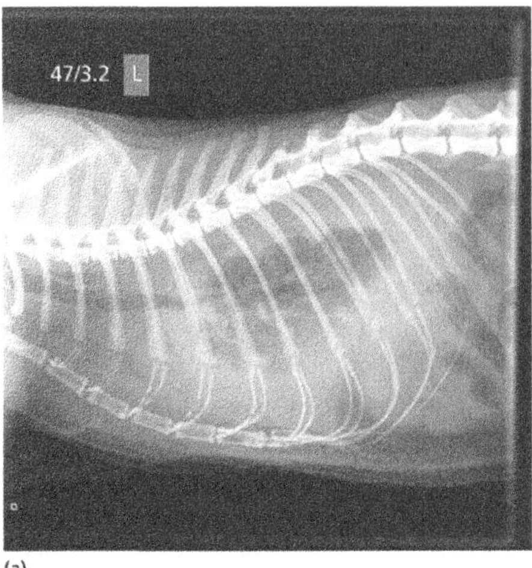

(a)

(b)

Figure 3.8 (a) X-ray showing marked retraction of the lung lobes due to pleural effusion. (b) Follow-up X-ray post-thoracocentesis showing poorly defined areas of soft tissue opacity, which could be inflammatory or neoplastic.

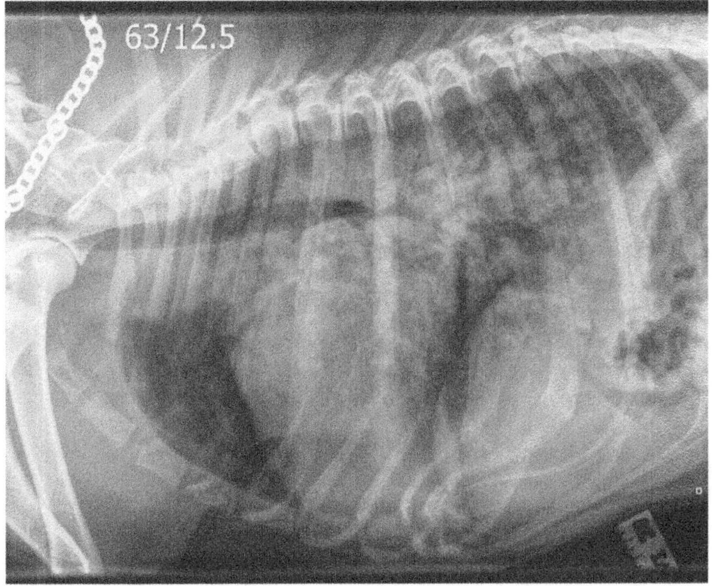

Figure 3.9 X-ray showing a left-sided cardiomegaly associated with severe pulmonary oedema.

high protein content, indicating infection, inflammation or malignancy (Kenyon & Kenyon, 2009).

Pulmonary oedema occurs when fluid accumulates in the lungs. It is often the result of left ventricular failure when a back pressure builds in the pulmonary veins causing fluid to be pushed from the veins into the alveoli (Figure 3.9). Pulmonary oedema may also occur with mitral or aortic valve damage, or fluid overload. Symptoms include dyspnoea, wheezing, tachycardia and coughing up white or pink-tinged frothy secretions (Kenyon & Kenyon, 2009).

CASE STUDY: PHYSIOTHERAPY TREATMENT PLAN FOR PNEUMONIA

Clinical history

Mojo is a 6-year-old female cross-breed. Her owner presented Mojo to the veterinary surgeon because Mojo was reluctant to exercise, and had developed a cough.

Clinical examination

Temperature: 40°C
Pulse rate: 100 bpm
Respiratory rate: 24 bpm
Weight: 25 kg
PMH: Nil of note. Mojo is up to date with vaccinations, worming and flea treatment. She has not travelled outside the UK.
HPC: Over the past 7–10 days Mojo has been reluctant to go for walks; she is eating less, sleeping more, and over the last few days she has developed a moist productive cough, which is most evident when she exerts herself.
DH: Nil at present.
SH: No other dogs in the household; Mojo has access to a large back garden.

Investigations

- CXR shows dilatation of the oesophagus; there is a mottled increased opacity over the ventral thorax with areas of alveolar pattern suggestive of pneumonia.
- ABGs show a decreased pH, increased P_aCO_2, normal HCO_3, indicating respiratory acidosis (uncompensated).

Diagnosis

- Pneumonia

Inpatient treatment

- Nebulise with normal saline every 4–6 hours.
- O_2 via nasal prongs 2 L/min humidified.

Medication

- Intravenous fluid therapy (IVFT), 1.5 × maintenance rate.
- Antibiotics: amoxicillin and clavulanic acid.

Physiotherapy respiratory assessment

- Review CXR and ABGs.
- Auscultation: breath sounds throughout, increased coarse crackles right mid-zone.
- SPO_2 94% on O_2 supplement as above.
- Increased respiratory rate (RR) ,with increased effort on inspiration.
- Observe position: patient positioned in sternal recumbency, with left hip down.
- Observe chest expansion: reduced expansion on righthand side.
- Observe cough: is it productive (volume, colour, consistency)? Productive cough, moderate (++) volume of mucopurulent, slightly discoloured, viscous fluid.
- Percussion note: dull over right mid-zone.

Physiotherapy

Day 1

Review HDU sheet and liaise with nursing staff for any relevant changes in the patient's condition.

Auscultate chest, compare left and right sides.

Obtain baseline measures for RR and SPO_2, prior to treatment to evaluate its effectiveness.

Mobilise patient 2 × 10 metres, with slings and harness if necessary; give the patient plenty of support and do not rush her.

Perform percussion to the affected area to encourage the patient to cough and clear secretions. If the patient expectorates observe colour, volume and consistency. Re-auscultate the chest; if *crackles* are still evident continue with percussion over the affected area to encourage the patient to cough and clear the secretions.

Measure RR and SPO_2 again and use these outcome measures to evaluate the effectiveness of the physiotherapy treatment. When treatment is successful the RR should decrease and the SPO_2 increase; however, be aware that these outcome measures will not return to *within normal limits* after a single physiotherapy treatment. Patients in the HDU or ICU would normally be seen for physiotherapy 3–4 times a day.

Position the patient in sternal recumbency, with the affected lung tilted slightly uppermost to aid postural drainage and for maximum ventilation. Position the unaffected lung in the dependent slightly downward position for maximum perfusion.

Maintain joint range of motion (ROM) with passive ROM (PROM) exercises 3 × 10 all limbs performed 2–3 times a day.

Maintain muscle length with passive protraction, retraction and internal rotator stretches, 3× with 15-second hold, performed 2–3 times a day.

Ask the HDU/ICU nursing staff to turn the patient's hips every 4 hours and place an adductor wedge between the pelvic limbs to maintain muscle length.

Remember to connect the patient back onto any intravenous fluids, or oxygen supplementation.

Communicate your findings to the multidisciplinary team (MDT) and write up treatment notes on the HDU/ICU sheet.

Day 2

Mobilise the patient 4 × 10 metres using support and assisting the patient as necessary.

Manual techniques: percussion over the affected area.

Position in sternal recumbency with a slight tilt to left.

Continue with PROM exercises and stretches three times daily.

Day 3

Mobilise 4 × 15 metres; increase the pace to encourage deep breaths and to increase lung volume. If the patient is able, reduce the support and assistance given and encourage her to support her own bodyweight.

Manual techniques: apply percussion over the affected area.

Positioning: she is now able to find her own independent position, and mobilise around the kennel, so it is not necessary to change hip position every 4 hours now.

Reduce PROM exercises and stretches to twice a day as the patient is becoming more mobile and less dependent.

Day 4

Mobilise 4 × 20 metres; increase pace to encourage deep breaths to increase lung volume, and begin to add in slopes to increase her stamina and strength.

The patient is now no longer on IVFT, O_2 or requiring nebulising. She is independently taking adequate oral fluids and eating well.

CXR much improved.

ABGs normal.

RR improved (reduced) 15 bpm.

SPO_2 improved at 98%.

Positioning: able to find own independent position.

Reduce PROM exercises and stretches to once a day as the patient is becoming more mobile and less dependent.

Other relevant conditions

Atelectasis

This is the term used to describe collapse of part of a lung, or occasionally the entire lung. It is caused by blockage of the bronchus or bronchioles.

Assessment findings (see Appendix 3)

- Reduced SPO_2: caused by a loss of lung volume.
- Auscultation: reduced breath sounds over the affected area as air cannot pass easily into that area, with late inspiratory crackles.
- Percussion note: is dull, due to reduced air entry into the affected area, and a loss of lung volume in that area.
- CXR: reduced lung volume, will show as an area of increased density.
- Chest palpation: reduced thoracic expansion, due to reduced functional lung capacity.

Physiotherapy management

- Mobilisation: this will encourage the patient to take deeper breaths and therefore increase air inspiration into the affected area of lung to increase lung volume.

- Position to optimise V/Q: if the left side is affected position the patient with this lung uppermost to improve ventilation, and the right lung down for maximum perfusion.
- Non-invasive ventilation (NIV): if the patient is struggling to maintain adequate SPO_2 levels non-invasive ventilation using nasal prongs should be considered.

Bronchospasm

This occurs when the airways constrict, and is often exercise induced.

Assessment (see Appendix 4)

- Reduced SPO_2: due to narrowed airways.
- Auscultation: expiratory wheeze is evident as the patient forces expired gases out of the narrowed airways.
- CXR: hyperinflation is often evident in chronic cases as the patient experiences increased work of breathing.
- Altered breathing pattern: the normal inspiration:expiration ratio will be altered, with a prolonged, active expiratory phase as the patient struggles to eliminate CO_2 through the narrow airways.

Physiotherapy management

- Positioning: often the upper lung lobes are affected and the patient may find it easier to rest and sleep in a supported sitting position, or at least resting in sternal recumbency with the head supported to prevent bronchospasm and to optimise ventilation.
- Bronchodilator therapy: such as salbutamol, which the veterinary surgeon may prescribe.

V/Q mismatch

This occurs when the patient has a reduced lung volume, which may be due to pneumonia, for example. If the patient is correctly positioned the affected lung can be adequately perfused and the opposing unaffected lung can be positioned in the dependent position to maximise lung perfusion.

Assessment (see Appendix 5)

- Reduced SPO_2: caused by the affected lung being perfused rather than ventilated.
- Auscultation: will demonstrate reduced breath sounds and late inspiratory crackles over the affected area, as reduced air flow is forced through the affected area.
- Percussion note: will be dull over the affected area as less air will flow to this region.
- CXR: volume loss or consolidation will show as an area of increased density.
- ABGs: may be altered and the patient may develop a respiratory acidosis with a decreased pH and increased P_aCO_2 with a normal HCO_3 in uncompensated patients. In chronic cases the patient may compensate for the respiratory acidosis and have a normal pH, with an increased P_aCO_2 and HCO_3.

Management

- Position to optimise V/Q: position and support the patient with the affected lung uppermost to maximise ventilation, and the unaffected lung down to maximise perfusion.
- Humidification and hydration: if the affected area is humidified and the patient hydrated he will find it easier to cough and clear secretions and therefore increase his lung volume. If the patient becomes dehydrated the affected area is likely to become consolidated making it more difficult for him to cough clear secretions to increase his lung volume.

Pain

It is important that postoperative patient pain is well managed; if not the patient's respiration may become compromised, especially so with cranial abdominal and thoracic surgery (see Appendix 6).

Assessment

- Reduced SPO_2: if the patient has altered respiratory function secondary to pain he may have a reduced SPO_2.
- Altered ABGs: if the patient is reluctant to breathe because of thoracic pain he may develop a respiratory acidosis, with a decreased pH, increased P_aCO_2 and normal HCO_3 if uncompensated. However, if he has an increased, shallow respiratory rate he may develop a respiratory alkalosis, with an increased pH, decreased P_aCO_2 and normal HCO_3 if uncompensated.
- Impaired cough: if the patient has abdominal or thoracic pain associated with recent surgery he will be reluctant to cough, and this could lead to retention of secretions if the pain is not controlled.
- Pain score: the patient should be pain scored to ensure he has adequate analgesia.

Management

- Pain management: a multi-modal approach should be adopted utilising local anaesthetic pain blocks when indicated, e.g. for chest drains.
- Positioning: use supports to position the patient so he is not putting excessive pressure on the painful site.
- Wound support: if the patient is attempting to cough and clear secretions, but his cough is weak due to pain, a folded towel can be placed over the incision site and a counter pressure applied to support the chest when the patient coughs to reduce excessive thoracic expansion and subsequent pain.

Hypoxaemia

Hypoxaemia is classified as a type I respiratory failure and is defined as $P_aO_2 < 60$ mmHg.

Assessment (see Appendix 7)

- Reduced SPO_2: due to inadequate gas exchange resulting in a decrease in P_aO_2.
- Mucous membrane colour: pale to cyanotic.
- Altered ABGs: in acute cases pH is decreased, P_aCO_2 is increased and HCO_3 is normal. In chronic cases pH may be normal, P_aCO_2 is increased and HCO_3 is increased.
- Altered Glasgow Coma Scale (GCS): due to inadequate gas exchange and a decrease in P_aO_2.

Management

- O_2 therapy/NIV: to correct the P_aO_2 deficit.
- Positioning: the patient may find standing, sitting or sternal recumbency with his head supported in neutral the most efficient position to maximise gas exchange. In such positions large areas of lung tissue will be ventilated.

N.B. Do not position an unstable hypoxic patient in dorsal recumbency even for a "quick" chest X-ray as he will experience V/Q mismatch, with the greatest lung surface area being perfused, rather than ventilated.

Self-assessment questions

1 When would manual techniques (percussion, vibrations, etc.) be contraindicated?

- **a** Pneumonia
- **b** Bronchitis
- **c** Pneumothorax
- **d** Retention of secretions.

2 Which of the following ABG results would indicate an uncompensated respiratory acidosis?

- **a** pH decreased; P_aCO_2 increased; HCO_3 normal.
- **b** pH increased; P_aCO_2 decreased; HCO_3 normal.

c pH decreased; P_aCO_2 normal; HCO_3 decreased.
d pH increased; P_aCO_2 normal; HCO_3 increased.

3 Which of the following ABG results would indicate a compensated respiratory acidosis?
a pH normal; P_aCO_2 increased; HCO_3 increased.
b pH increased; P_aCO_2 decreased; HCO_3 normal.
c pH decreased; P_aCO_2 normal; HCO_3 decreased.
d pH increased; P_aCO_2 normal; HCO_3 increased.

4 What is a normal inspiratory/expiratory respiratory ratio?
a 2:1
b 1:1
c 2:2
d 1:2

5 In a patient with COPD how would this inspiratory/expiratory ratio change?
a 2:2
b 1:2
c 2:3
d 1:3

6 When auscultating a chest which condition would you associate with fine end-of-inspiration crackles?
a Pleural effusion
b Emphysema
c Bronchitis
d Pulmonary oedema.

7 Which of the following conditions would benefit from manual physiotherapy techniques (percussion and vibrations)?
a Pleural effusion
b Emphysema
c Bronchitis
d Pulmonary oedema.

8 Which of the following conditions is not classified as COPD?
a Bronchitis
b Asthma
c Pneumonia
d Emphysema.

9 Which of the following equations measures cardiac output (CO)?
a CO = HR/SV
b CO = MAP × HR
c CO = HR × SV
d CO = MAP × SV

10 Which of the following is used to measure hypoxia?
a pH
b P_aO_2
c P_aCO_2
d HCO_3

CHAPTER 4
Hydrotherapy

Introduction

Hydrotherapy allows the animal to exercise in water. The properties of water can provide an ideal environment to assist weak animals to regain motor function, or in the more able animal water can be used to provide resistance and have a muscle-strengthening effect.

The aims of hydrotherapy

Maintain or improve joint ROM

When an animal is exercising in a water treadmill and lifts his limb to propel himself forwards the buoyancy effect of the water will further increase flexion of the limbs joints.

Improve muscle strengthening

The density and gravity of the animal in water and the resistance from the viscosity of the water molecules will provide the animal with an ideal environment in which to exercise and improve muscle

---

Practical Physiotherapy for Veterinary Nurses, First Edition. Donna Carver.

strength. To progress the patient use less water so reducing the buoyancy effect of the water and focusing on strengthening as the animal navigates against the resistance provided by the water. Further resistance can be added by using water jets for the animal to work against.

Gait re-education

The water will provide support for animals with neurological conditions and balance deficits. If these animals are recovering from spinal surgery they may need to re-learn motor movement patterns. A water treadmill is an ideal environment as the level of the water can be controlled to maximise the buoyancy effect from the water; also, the speed of the treadmill belt can be controlled to allow the animal extra time for voluntary motor function in the affected limbs. Moreover, the therapist will be in the water with the patient so she or he will be able to passively assist the patient to move his affected limbs in a functional pattern, when the patient is supported with a buoyancy jacket, sling and an over-treadmill hoist.

Reduce pain

The warmth of the water can reduce muscle tension and associated pain from trigger points allowing the patient to exercise in a comfortable environment. The hydrostatic pressure from the water can reduce pain in arthritic patients with swollen joints, and the buoyancy effect of the water ensures less bodyweight is passing through these joints and therefore reduces the concussive forces passing through the joints, so that the animal is able to exercise in a comfortable environment and therefore build muscle to support and stabilise the painful joints.

Improve stamina

The viscosity or resistance properties of water can be used to improve cardiovascular fitness and stamina. The duration of time exercising in the water treadmill can gradually be increased, with the rest intervals being gradually decreased. As the patient progresses the speed of the belt can also be increased. Finally, adding in resistance with water jets will improve stamina and strength.

Pool chemistry

A pool tester kit should be used to check the pH and bromine levels in the water storage tank *at least once a day*, or more frequently if the water is becoming contaminated between patients. The pH should be adjusted first, followed by the bromine.

Personnel must take care when handling these chemicals by wearing protective gloves to prevent skin irritation, protective googles to protect the eyes from splashes, and a face mask to prevent the chemicals from being inhaled.

pH

The pH of the water is an indication of the acidity or alkalinity of water. The pH should be maintained between 7.2 and 7.6; when the water becomes contaminated with bacteria the pH will fall and the water will become more acidic. Aqua Sparkle Spa pH Plus (PoolMarket.co.uk, Bristol, UK) can be added when the level falls below 7.2, Aqua Sparkle Spa pH Minus (PoolMarket.co.uk, Bristol, UK) should be added to the storage tank if the level rises above 7.6. Ensure that any added pH powder is well mixed with the water in the storage tank.

Bromine

Bromine is a chemical similar to chlorine used in swimming pools to prevent the water from becoming contaminated with bacteria. When the water becomes contaminated with bacteria the level of bromine will fall; the level of bromine should be maintained between 2 and 6 ppm (parts per million). Small quantities of bromine powder can be added to boost the level should the level drop below 2 ppm.

Bromine tablets are also available, which slowly dissolve over a period of weeks in the tank to maintain a baseline bromine level within the storage tank.

Temperature

The water should be maintained at a comfortable temperature for the animal to exercise in. A temperature of 30°C is recommended to reduce muscle tension or spasm and to provide the patient with optimum conditions to exercise in.

Properties of water

Density

The density of an object is the ratio of the weight of the object relative to an equal volume of water (Haralson, 1988). Densities of various substances are defined by their specific gravity; the specific gravity of water is 1.0. The density and specific gravity of an object will determine how well it will float. If the ratio of the object's specific gravity to that of water is greater than 1, the object will tend to sink, and if less than 1 the object will tend to float (Edlich et al., 1987).

A lean animal will have a higher specific gravity than water, and will be less buoyant in water than an obese animal, which will have a specific gravity lower than the water; hence the obese animal will tend to be more buoyant in water and float.

Buoyancy

A body immersed in water will experience two opposing forces: gravity is the downward force, while buoyancy is the upward thrust of water acting on a body that creates an apparent decrease in the weight of the body while immersed (Hecox et al., 1994).

Weak animals can benefit from buoyancy as the weight passing through the limbs will be less, so the weak animal may find it easier to move and exercise in water. The same principles would apply to animals with painful joints: the buoyancy effect would result in less bodyweight and lower concussive forces passing through the joints, so the animal would be more comfortable exercising in water.

Viscosity

The viscosity of water, or its resistance, is significantly greater than that of air. The resistance from water can be used to strengthen muscles in animals and therefore support the joints, and also to improve cardiovascular fitness and stamina. The viscosity of the water can be used to increase support in neurological patients who may have significant balance deficits on dry land.

Hydrostatic pressure

The deeper the body is immersed in water the greater the hydrostatic pressure exerted on it. This pressure can be advantageous to animals with peripheral tissue oedema or swollen joints, such as arthritic patients, because the water pressure will exert a force on these tissues to gently reduce the tissue oedema and swelling around painful joints.

Water surface tension

Water molecules have a greater tendency to adhere together on the surface. Resistance to movement is slightly greater on the surface of water because there is more cohesion on the surface of the water (Hecox et al., 1994). Keep this in mind when setting the level of water for the patient to exercise in, and ensure the level and therefore surface tension of water corresponds to the muscle groups to be strengthened.

Hydrotherapy for specific conditions

Hydrotherapy can be a very useful modality in the rehabilitation of neurological patients, who will benefit from the buoyancy effect provided by the water. The buoyancy of the patient can be further enhanced by using flotation equipment such as buoyancy jackets. Very weak patients should also be fitted with a neck support float as they may find it difficult to maintain head control in the early rehabilitation stages.

It is vital that a trained member of staff goes into the water with paraparetic or tetraparetic patients to reassure them should they panic, and to assist them with movement of the affected limbs and support the patient as necessary. Paraparetic patients should be supported with a Helping Hand or The Soft Quick Lift™ sling attached to a hoist; this allows the person in the water with the patient to use their hands to facilitate movement of the patient's affected weak limbs. A second person should be poolside at all times to assist as necessary.

Tetraparetic patients should be supported with a body sling attached to a hoist with two people available to assist the patient at all times; at least one person needs to be in the water with the patient to ensure patient safety and to assist the patient as necessary.

Remember that neurological patients will tire very quickly: even being supported in stance with a body sling whist the water chamber of an underwater treadmill (UWT) fills or empties can be enough to tire these patients in the early rehabilitation stages. Keep the sessions short, provide plenty of rest breaks, give the patient maximum support and utilise buoyancy aids and flotation devices.

After the hydrotherapy session remember to shampoo the patient to wash bromine from his coat, and dry him well so he does not become cold. If he is returning to the ward make sure he is correctly positioned, so that weak limbs are supported, and that he is kept covered with blankets and comfortably warm.

If spinal patients begin hydrotherapy before skin sutures or staples have been removed use a waterproof dressing to protect this area. When to start hydrotherapy in these patients will be at the discretion of the veterinary surgeon, and also depend on the confidence of the staff that carry out the hydrotherapy for this group of patients.

CASE STUDY: HEMILAMINECTOMY INTERVERTEBRAL DISC DECOMPRESSION T13-L1 DAY 5 POSTOPERATIVE HYDROTHERAPY REHABILITATION PROGRAMME

History

Rocco is a 7-year-old Staffordshire bull terrier; 5 days post hemilaminectomy intervertebral disc decompression (HLE IVDD) at the level of T13 – L1.

Rocco mobilises with a Helping Hand sling and moderate assistance from one person. Foot protectors are used to prevent scuffing and damage to the dorsal aspect of the paws. He has weak pelvic limb (PL) voluntary motor function (VMF): hip > stifle > hock; he is not placing his PLs. His owner reports he is used to paddling in water but he does not go in deep or swim.

First hydrotherapy session

- Cover the surgical site with a waterproof dressing.
- Fit with a buoyancy jacket, ensuring a snug fit for maximum buoyancy.
- Walk the patient into the treadmill supporting his PLs with a sling.
- Attach the handles of the sling to the hoist and adjust the height so that the patient's PLs are lightly resting in the middle of the treadmill belt.
- Reassure him as necessary.
- Begin to fill the UWT chamber with water heated to 30°C to the level of the patient's mid-thorax; ensure the water is not too close to the patient's face as he may panic.
- One person should be poolside to support and guide the patient on the treadmill belt; the second person is in the water with the patient to support him, reassure him, and also to facilitate functional movement in the affected weak limbs.
- Remember to allow plenty of time for VMF in the weak limbs; set the speed of the belt slower than the patient's normal walking speed to allow for weak PL VMF.
- Assist the patient to flex and place his PLs by applying a forward pressure behind the caudal aspect of the stifles in time to facilitate a reciprocal gait pattern; that is, as he steps forwards with his right thoracic limb (TL) assist him to step forwards with his left PL, then when he steps forwards with his left TL assist him to step forwards on his right PL to facilitate a normal reciprocal gait pattern.

Progression

As the patient progresses the time exercising and speed of the treadmill belt can be increased to improve fitness and stamina, and also to encourage greater stride length and joint range of motion (ROM). The support given to the patient in the water can be reduced, and also the buoyancy effect can be reduced by lowering the level of the water to focus on strengthening the patient. Water jets can also be added to further strengthen the patient as he has to work against resistance. Finally, the water will also support the patient, so when the level of water is reduced this will also challenge and improve his balance (see Video 4.1).

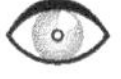

VIDEO 4.1

Hemilaminectomy outpatient hydrotherapy. The patient is weak in his pelvic limbs; he shows occasional *knuckling* on his pelvic limbs indicating reduced proprioception. The water jets are used to further strengthen the patient as he works against resistance.

Fibrocartilage embolism hydrotherapy rehabilitation programme

Post-fibrocartilage embolism (FCE) patients often present for hydrotherapy. The aim of the hydrotherapy is to strengthen the affected limb(s), and improve joint ROM, cardiovascular (CV) fitness, balance and proprioception to return the patient to his highest level of function.

Generally non-surgical FCE patient rehabilitation tends to be more vigorous as there is no healing surgical site or surgical interventions to take into consideration. Early progress in FCE patients is often linked to a more favourable prognosis. However, the patient will still need support in the water and plenty of reassurance as he will feel vulnerable in the early stages in the water. Keep the sessions short to begin with and use the buoyancy effect of the water to give him support. Set the speed of the treadmill belt slower than his normal walking speed to allow extra time for VMF in the affected limbs. Assist the patient as necessary to flex and place his affected limbs using a functional gait pattern.

The goals of the hydrotherapy sessions are to progressively:

- Improve joint ROM.
- Improve muscle strength and core stability.
- Improve balance and proprioception.
- Improve CV fitness.

Joint ROM in the limbs will be greater than when exercising on dry land as the buoyancy effect of the water will increase flexion of the limbs. When assisting the patient in his weak affected limbs, ROM of the joints should also be exaggerated to reinforce normal movement patterns.

Muscle strength will improve when the patient is actively exercising in the UWT. As the patient progresses water levels can be reduced to provide resistance to the patient, and further resistance can be added by incorporating the use of water jets. When navigating his way through the water and resistance he will also engage his core muscles, and begin to strengthen these.

The patient's balance and proprioception will be challenged when the water level is lowered, as he will be less supported.

The speed of the belt and duration of time spent exercising with reduced rest time will improve the patient's CV fitness.

Remember to start slow and offer lots of support and assistance in the early phase of the rehabilitation programme. The focus of the early programme will be to facilitate VMF, and improve joint ROM. As the patient progresses into the mid-phase of the rehabilitation programme he will become more confident and need less assistance; aim to improve his strength, balance and proprioception in this phase.

In the late phase of the programme focus on improving the patient's CV fitness to rehabilitate him to his highest level of function (see 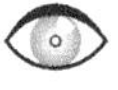 Videos 4.2 and 4.3).

VIDEO 4.2

Fibrocartilage embolism (FCE) gait. The video show a patient at 6 weeks post-FCE. The patient is monoparetic and ataxic in the left pelvic limb. Weakness in the affected limb can be observed as she adopts a *crab-like sideways walking* pattern, and when she increases her pace she *bunnyhops*. She has a high-stepping gait pattern in the affected limb typically seen in ataxic patients.

VIDEO 4.3

Fibrocartilage embolism (FCE) hydrotherapy gait. This video was taken on the same day as Video 4.2 and shows the same patient exercising in the underwater treadmill. Note the reduced ataxia in the affected limb. With the pace controlled and with the support of the water the patient's gait pattern is much improved.

CASE STUDY: OSTEOARTHRITIS HYDROTHERAPY REHABILITATION PROGRAMME

History

Max is a 6-year-old male boxer diagnosed by his veterinary surgeon with hip dysplasia and secondary osteoarthritis. He intermittently takes non-steroidal anti-inflammatory drugs (NSAIDs) when he has a flare-up of pain (often associated with over-exercise); he also takes glucosamine and chondroitin joint supplements. His bodyweight is ideal; he has 2 × 15 minute lead walks and 2 × 30 minute off-lead walks a day. He presented to his veterinary surgeon as he was stiff to rise in the morning. On physical examination the veterinary surgeon noted reduced hip extension with pain at end of range, and reduced muscle bulk on the pelvic limbs. He has been referred for hydrotherapy to improve pelvic limb muscle bulk and strength.

Physiotherapy assessment

Gait: Short stride length, reduced hip extension and internal rotation of right hip joint. 1-2/5 lame right pelvic limb at trot.

Joint ROM: Reduced bilateral hip extension and abduction; right limb more affected than left. Right pelvic limb extension 145°, left pelvic limb extension 150°.

Muscle mass: Reduced bulk pelvic limbs, right more affected than left. Right pelvic limb 30 cm, left pelvic limb 34 cm.

Muscle length: Slightly tight bilateral hamstrings.

Weight-bearing through limbs: Shifts weight from right to left pelvic limb in stance: right pelvic limb 45%, left pelvic limb 55%; right thoracic limb 48%, left thoracic limb 52%.

Secondary compensatory issues: Increased muscle tension over lumbar spine with *trigger points* evident.

Problem list

1 Pain/altered gait pattern.
2 Reduced joint ROM.
3 Reduced muscle mass.
4 Secondary lumbar spine muscle tension.

Goals

1 Reduce pain/gait re-education (2–12 weeks).
2 Improve joint ROM (6 weeks).
3 Improve muscle mass (6 weeks).
4 Reduce secondary compensatory issues (6 weeks).

Treatment plan

The hydrotherapy plan below would assume the patient was seen once per week. At 6 weeks evaluate his progress comparing the outcome measures obtained with the baseline assessment measures. If the patient is making steady progress at week 6, the next six hydrotherapy sessions can be gradually progressed in terms of speed, time and resistance to return the patient to his highest functional level, and to ensure the list of goals drawn up from the assessment findings have been met.

First hydrotherapy session

The temperature of the water is set to 30°C. This is a comfortable temperature for the patient to exercise in; the warmth of the water will help to reduce muscle tension. The patient is fitted with a snug buoyancy jacket to ensure that less bodyweight is passing through the arthritic joints.

The water level is set to the proximal femur; again this is to take advantage of the buoyancy effect of the water and assist the patient with his early hydrotherapy exercise programme. The speed of the treadmill belt is set at 4 kph; this is actually slightly slower than the patient's normal walking speed, but is selected so he can become used to exercising in the water.

The duration of the first hydrotherapy session is kept short at 3 × 1 minutes of exercise. Remember, if this is the first time the patient has exercised in water this way he may become anxious so short sessions are preferable in the early stages. Again a work/rest ratio of 1:1 is recommended for the early sessions to allow the patient to become accustomed to the new environment and exercise programme.

Second hydrotherapy session

Assuming the patient is comfortable continue with the first hydrotherapy session programme, *but*: increase the exercise time to 4 × 1 minutes.

Third hydrotherapy session

Assuming the patient is comfortable continue with the second hydrotherapy session programme, *but*: increase the treadmill belt speed to 5 kph.

Fourth hydrotherapy session

Assuming the patient is comfortable continue with the third hydrotherapy session programme, *but*: alter the work/rest ratio to 2:1. 2 minutes work, with 1 minute rest, repeat 4 times.

Fifth hydrotherapy session

Assuming the patient is comfortable continue with the fourth hydrotherapy session programme, *but*: add in resistance from the water jets to the exercise programme.

Sixth hydrotherapy session

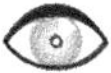

Assuming the patient is comfortable continue with the fifth hydrotherapy session programme, *but*: reduce the level of the water to mid-femur (see Video 4.4).

Evaluation and outcome measures

- Evaluate pain and lameness score plus subjective feedback from owner.
- Measure the percentage of weight-bearing through limbs; compare with assessment baseline measures.
- Measure joint ROM with a goniometer and compare with assessment baseline measures.
- Measure pelvic limb global muscle mass around the circumference of the limb at the level of the quadriceps and hamstrings muscle belly. Compare with assessment baseline measures.
- Measuring respiratory and heart rate pre- and post-exercise will give an indication of the patient's CV fitness and stamina levels. As the patient progresses his respiratory and heart rate following exercise may decrease, from the original baseline measures meaning he is able to exercise at a higher intensity.

Progression

- As the patient improves and if pain is under control, start to progress the hydrotherapy programme.
- The *speed* of the treadmill belt can be increased; this will encourage the patient to take a longer stride, therefore increasing joint ROM. Increasing the speed of the treadmill belt will also improve the patient's CV fitness.
- The *buoyancy* effect is not as necessary once the patient begins to progress, and if he remains pain free the *level of the water* can be adjusted so that he has to push through the *surface tension* of the water as he is exercising to improve muscle mass and strength. Further strengthening can be achieved by using resistance from water jets.
- The *duration* of time spend exercising in the UWT can be increased, and the *rest time* between exercising can be decreased to improve stamina.

Patient discharge

If the goals that were drawn up at assessment have been met at 12 weeks consider discharging the patient, or if the owner prefers, reduce the hydrotherapy sessions to once every 2 weeks, or once every 4 weeks. Outcome measures recorded at baseline and at 6 weeks should be repeated again at 12 weeks to evaluate progress and to inform the referring veterinary surgeon of the patient's progress.

Owner education for their pet would focus on encouraging regular gentle exercise, and the use of supportive bedding.

VIDEO 4.4

Hip dysplasia outpatient hydrotherapy. The video shows a patient with hip dysplasia whose right pelvic limb is more affected than the left. Note the patient does not wear a buoyancy jacket as he is well behaved and he is working to strengthen the muscles of the pelvic limbs to support the hip joint. The right hip joint is slightly internally rotated, and reduced limb stability can be seen with pelvic rotation.

CASE STUDY: PELVIC LIMB AMPUTATION HYDROTHERAPY REHABILITATION PROGRAMME

History

Jasmine is a 9-year-old bull mastiff referred for hydrotherapy 4 weeks post-right pelvic limb amputation.

Assessment

Gait: Ambulatory, weak on left pelvic limb due to overload; owner uses a sling to assist Jasmine with balance and to provide additional support when she tires.
Posture: Slight rotation of lumbo-sacral (L-S) spine following right pelvic limb amputation (due to weakness).
Joint ROM: Functional in remaining three limbs. Slight stiffness and reduced flexion bilateral elbows; some thickening of elbow joints.
Muscle mass: Increased muscle tension left pelvic limb.
Muscle length: Functional.
Secondary compensatory issues: Increased muscle tension in left pelvic limb, and L-S spine rotation due to weakness post-amputation.

Problem list

1. Altered gait pattern.
2. Reduced joint ROM (elbows).
3. Increased muscle tension left PL.
4. Secondary postural changes (L-S) spine.
5. Reduced strength.

6 Reduced balance.
7 Reduced stamina.

Goals

1 Gait re-education (2–12 weeks).
2 Improve joint ROM (6 weeks).
3 Reduce muscle tension (6 weeks).
4 Reduce secondary postural issues (6 weeks).
5 Improve strength (6–12 weeks).
6 Improve balance (6–12 weeks).
7 Improve stamina (6–12 weeks).

Treatment

First hydrotherapy session

Use a snug-fitting buoyancy jacket to give maximum support in the water. Ensure a member of staff goes into the water with the patient to reassure her, should she panic. A second person should remain poolside to guide the patient on the treadmill belt. Keep the first session short, with plenty of rest breaks. Set the treadmill belt speed slightly slower than the patient's normal gait speed so she can become accustomed to the new exercise environment.

Second hydrotherapy session

The aim of the second session is to improve the patient's gait pattern; the water will give her support so less weight will be passing through the left pelvic limb, and therefore her L-S spine should be less rotated and the patient will have improved posture/spinal alignment.

Third hydrotherapy session

The patient should at this point be accustomed to the new exercise environment. The warmth of the water will provide a pleasant exercise environment and may assist in reducing muscle tension in the left pelvic limb. The concussive forces passing through the elbow joints will be less in the water treadmill so the patient may be willing to exercise for longer in the water as opposed to exercising on dry land.

Fourth hydrotherapy session

As the patient continues to progress in terms of strength and speed, she will need less support in the water. The time spent exercising can be increased and the rest time can be reduced. The speed of the belt can also be increased to improve stride length and stamina.

Fifth hydrotherapy session

As the patient progresses and gains strength and confidence the water level can be reduced so the patient will need to work harder as she will have less buoyancy/support. By lowering the water her balance will also be challenged and so improve over time.

Sixth hydrotherapy session

At this stage the speed of the belt can be increased further; time exercising can also be increased, support decreased, and resistance from water jets added to further improve strength and stamina.

Evaluation and outcome measures

- Video the gait pattern and obtain subjective feedback from the owner; compare with baseline measures obtained at the initial assessment.
- Measure elbow joint ROM with a goniometer and compare with assessment baseline measures.
- Measuring respiratory and heart rates pre- and post-exercise will give an indication of the patient's CV fitness and stamina levels. As the patient progresses her respiratory and heart rates following exercise may decrease, (compared with original baseline measures), meaning she is able to exercise at a higher intensity (Figure 4.1 and Table 4.1).

Discharge

Repeat measures taken at assessment (baseline measures) and compare to evaluate patient progress at 6 weeks. If the patient has progressed to her highest level of function, discharge the patient with owner advice on a maintenance land exercise programme, and provide a discharge letter to the referring veterinary surgeon. Alternatively, it may be agreed with the owner that the patient continues to attend hydrotherapy to maintain fitness levels, attending once every 2 or 4 weeks.

If the patient has not achieved all of the goals drawn up from the problem list it may be that the patient needs to continue for another six weekly hydrotherapy sessions, after which outcome measures are repeated at week 12 to evaluate progress. If a patient deteriorates take the hydrotherapy session back a step, that is, reduce time/speed to assess if the patient is just fatigued; if the patient has really deteriorated consider referring the patient back to her referring vet to ensure that no further complications have arisen.

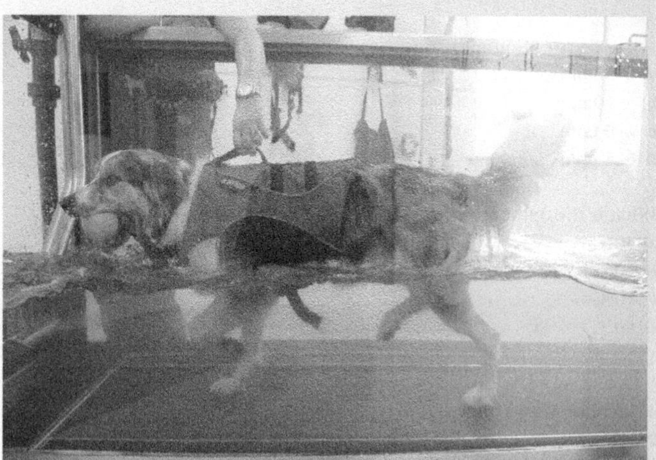

Figure 4.1 Patient with left thoracic limb biceps tendinopathy exercising in the underwater treadmill to strengthen the biceps muscle. Additional resistance is provided by the patient working against resistance from the water jets.

Table 4.1 Hydrotherapy progression.

Stamina/CV fitness	Balance	Strength
Increase time exercising	Reduce water level	Reduce buoyancy
Increase belt speed	Reduce buoyancy	Reduce water level
Reduce rest breaks	Reduce assistance	Reduce assistance
		Increase resistance (water jets)

Self-assessment questions

1 What is the optimum hydrotherapy pool pH level range?
  a 7.0–8.0
  b 8.2–8.6
  c 7.0–7.2
  d 7.2–7.6

2 What is the optimum hydrotherapy pool bromine level range?
  a 0–5 ppm
  b 5–10 ppm
  c 2–6 ppm
  d 6–8 ppm

3 What is the optimum hydrotherapy pool temperature?
  a 30°C
  b 20°C.
  c 10°C
  d 40°C

4 When using a UWT which variable should be adjusted to increase stride length?
  a Increase water level.
  b Decrease water level.
  c Increase treadmill belt speed.
  d Decrease treadmill belt speed.

5 Which variable will increase the patient's buoyancy when using a UWT?
  a Increasing resistance using water jets.
  b Decreasing resistance by not using water jets.
  c Decreasing the water level.
  d Increasing the water level.

6 When using a UWT at what level is there most resistance from the water?
  a At the surface level of the water.
  b 10 cm below the surface level of the water.
  c 20 cm below the surface level of the water.
  d 30 cm below the surface level of the water.

7 When treating a patient with hip dysplasia, at what level should the water be set to optimise patient strength?

a At the level of the tarsus.
b At the level of the stifle.
c At the level of the proximal femur.
d At the level above the hip joint.

8 When treating a patient with elbow dysplasia, at what level should the water be set to optimise patient strength?

a At the level of the shoulder joint.
b At the level just above the elbow joint.
c At the level of mid-radius.
d At the level of the carpus.

9 Which one of the following would be considered a caution when carrying out hydrotherapy in a UWT?

a The patient has a grade II heart murmur; he is not currently on any medication for this.
b It is the patient's first session and he is not used to deep water.
c The patient is sensitive to cold water.
d The owner does not know if the patient can swim.

10 Which one of the following would not be considered a contraindication when carrying out hydrotherapy in a UWT?

a The patient has an open discharging wound.
b The patient is incontinent.
c The patient has a skin infection.
d The patient has had sutures removed from a healed surgical incision site the day before.

APPENDICES

Appendix 1: Glasgow Coma Scale (GCS)

Eye opening		Best motor response		Best verbal response	
Spontaneous	4	Obeys commands	6	Orientated and vocal	5
To sound	3	Localises to pain	5	Disorientated and vocal	4
To pain	2	Flexion withdrawal to pain	4	Inappropriately vocalises	3
No response	1	Abnormal flexion	3	Inappropriate sounds	2
		Extension	2	No response	1
		No response	1		

Total score: 3 to 15.

Practical Physiotherapy for Veterinary Nurses, First Edition. Donna Carver.

Appendix 2: Secretion retention assessment and management plan

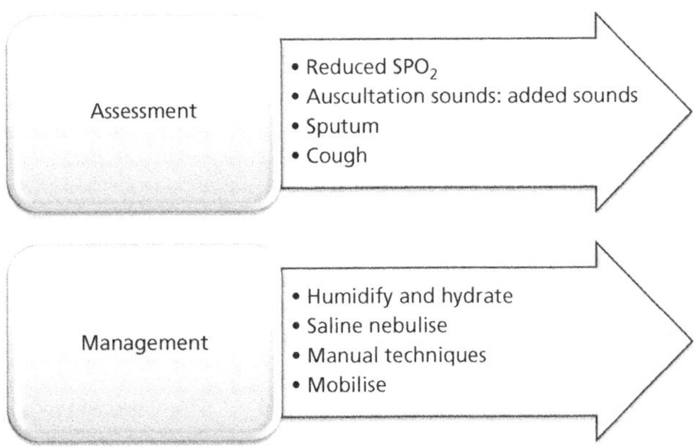

Appendix 3: Atelectasis assessment and management plan

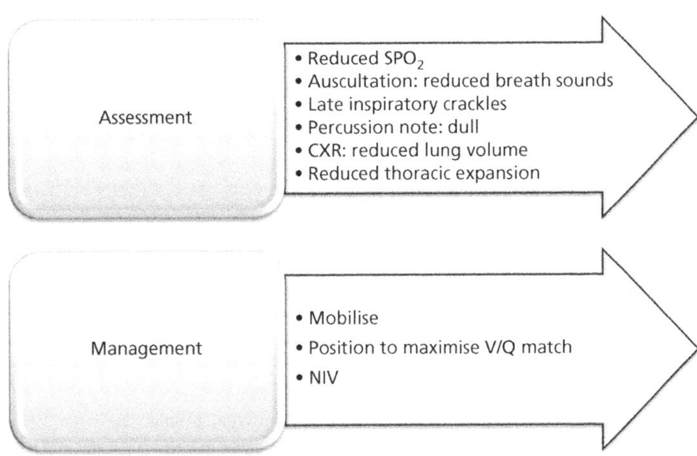

Appendix 4: Bronchospasm assessment and management plan

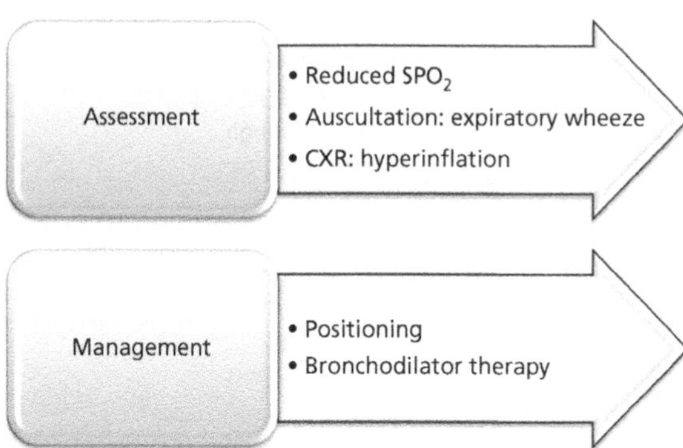

Appendix 5: V/Q mismatch assessment and management plan

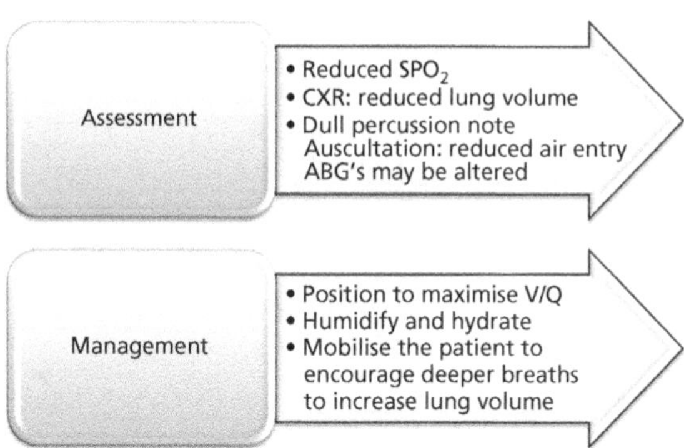

Appendix 6: Pain assessment and management plan

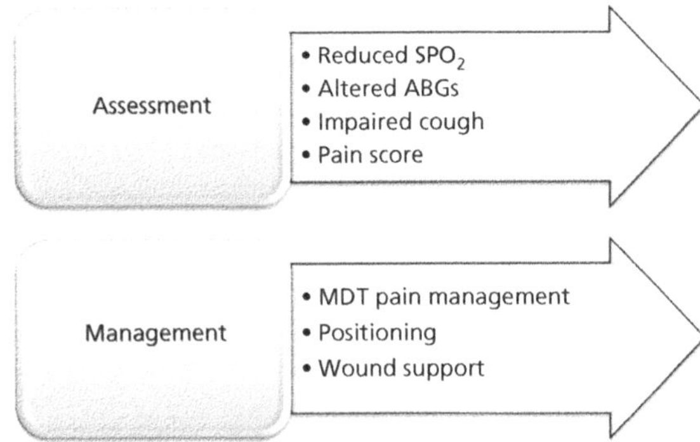

Appendix 7: Hypoxaemia assessment and management plan

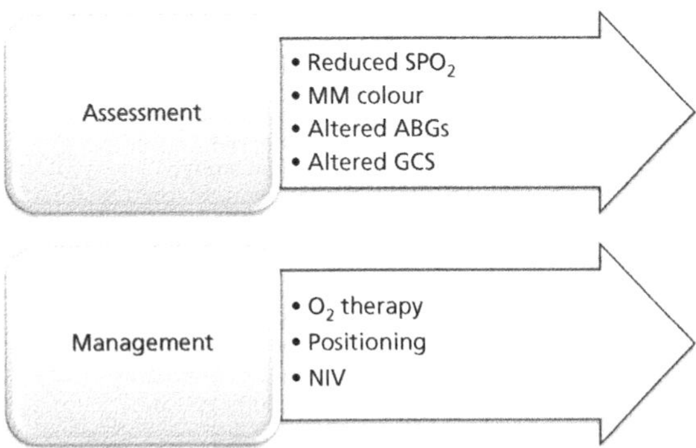

Abbreviations

ABG	Arterial blood gas
ABP	Arterial blood pressure
AS	Added sounds
BE	Base excess
BP	Blood pressure
bpm	Beats or breaths per minute
BSTO	Breath sounds throughout
°C	Degrees Celsius
CCL	Cranial cruciate ligament
CO	Cardiac output
CO_2	Carbon dioxide
COPD	Chronic obstructive pulmonary disease
CP	Conscious proprioception
CPP	Cerebral perfusion pressure
CT	Computed tomography
CVP	Central venous pressure
CXR	Chest X-ray
DH	Drug history
°F	Degrees Fahrenheit
FCE	Fibrocartilage embolism
FHNE	Femoral head and neck excision
FMCD	Fragmented medial coronoid disease
FWB	Full weight-bearing
GCMPS-SF	Glasgow Composite Measure Pain Scale – Short Form
GCS	Glasgow Coma Scale
HCO_3	Bicarbonate
HD	Hip dysplasia
HDU	High dependency unit
HR	Heart rate
ICP	Intracranial pressure
ICU	Intensive care unit
I:E	Inspiration:expiration ratio
IOHC	Incomplete ossification of humeral condyle
IVFT	Intravenous fluid therapy
kPa	Kilopascal

Practical Physiotherapy for Veterinary Nurses, First Edition. Donna Carver.

LHS Lefthand side
MAP Mean arterial pressure
MDT Multi-disciplinary team
mmHg Millimetres of mercury
NIV Non-invasive ventilation
O_2 Oxygen
OCD Osteochondritis dissecans
ORIF Open reduction internal fixation
OTT Over-the-top technique
PEME Pulsed electromagnetic energy
pH Potential of hydrogen (acid–alkali balance)
P_ACO_2 Partial pressure of carbon dioxide in blood
P_aCO_2 Partial pressure of carbon dioxide in arterial blood
P_aO_2 Partial pressure of oxygen in arterial blood
ppm Parts per million
PRICE Protection Rest Ice Compression Elevation
NSAID Non-steroidal anti-inflammatory drug
NWB Non-weight-bearing
PC Presenting condition
PL Pelvic limb
PMH Past medical history
PROM Passive range of motion
PUPD Polydipsia polyuria
PWB Partial weight-bearing
RHS Righthand side
ROM Range of motion
RR Respiratory rate
SH Social history
SIN Severity irritability nature
SPO_2 Peripheral capillary oxygen saturation
STR Soft tissue release
SV Stroke volume
SVR Stroke volume resistance
TENS Transcutaneous electrical nerve stimulation
THR Total hip replacement
TL Thoracic limb
TPLO Tibial plateau levelling osteotomy
TTA Tibial tuberosity advancement
TTO Triple tibial osteotomy
TWO Tibial wedge osteotomy
UAP Un-united anconeal process
UWT Underwater treadmill
VAS Visual analogue scale
VMF Voluntary motor function
V/Q Ventilation/perfusion
< Less than
> More than

References

Beal, B.S. (2004) Use of nutraceuticals and chondroprotectants in osteoarthritic dogs. *Veterinary Clinics of North America: Small Animal Practice* **34,** 271–289.

Beren, J., Hill, S.L., Diener-West, M., et al. (2001) The effect of preloading oral glucosamine/chondroitin sulfate/manganese ascorbate combination on experimental arthritis in rats. *Experimental Biology and Medicine* **226,** 144–152.

Binz, T., Sikorra, S. & Mahrhold, S. (2010) Clostridial neurotoxins: mechanisms of SNARE cleavage and outlook on potential substrate specificity reengineering. *Toxins (Basel)* **2,** 665–682.

Canapp, S.O., McLaughlin, R.M., Hoskinson, J.J., et al. (1999) Scintographic evaluation of glucosamine HCL and chondroitin sulfate as treatment for acute synovitis in dogs. *American Journal of Veterinary Research* **60,** 1552–1557.

Cauzinille, L. & Kornegay, J.N. (1996) Fibrocartilaginous embolism of the spinal cord in dogs: review of 36 historically confirmed cases and retrospective study of 26 suspected cases. *Journal of Veterinary Internal Medicine* **10,** 241–245.

Cummings, J.F. & Haas, D.C. (1966) Coonhound paralysis. An acute idiopathic polyradiculoneuritis in dogs resembling the Landry-Guillain-Barré syndrome. *Journal of Neurological Science* **4,** 51–81.

Edlich, R.F., Towler, M.A., Goitz, R.J., et al. (1987) Bioengineering principles of hydrotherapy. *Journal of Burn Care and Rehabilitation* **8,** 580–584.

Gandini, G., Cizinauskas, S., Lang, J., Fatzer, R. & Jaggy, A. (2003) Fibrocartilage embolism in 75 dogs: clinical findings and factors influencing the recovery rate. *Journal of Small Animal Practice* **44,** 76–80.

Haralson, K.M. (1998) Therapeutic pool programs. *Journal of Clinical Outcomes Management* **5,** 579–584.

Hecox, B., Mehreteab, T.A. & Weisberg, J. (1994) *Physical agents: a comprehensive text for physical therapists.* Appleton & Lange, Norwalk, CT.

Practical Physiotherapy for Veterinary Nurses, First Edition. Donna Carver.

Holt, N., Murray, M., Cuddon, P.A. & Lappin, M.R. (2011) Seroprevalence of various infectious agents in dogs with suspected acute polyradiculoneuritis. *Journal of Veterinary Internal Medicine* **25,** 261–266.

Hulse, D.S. (1998) Treatment methods for pain in the osteoarthritic patient. *Veterinary Clinics of North America: Small Animal Practice* **28,** 361–375.

Jefferey, N.D. & Blakemore, W.F. (1999) Spinal cord injury in small animals 1. Mechanisms of spontaneous recovery. *Veterinary Record* **144,** 407–413.

Kenyon, K. & Kenyon, J. (2009) *The physiotherapist's pocket book: essential facts at your fingertips*, 2nd edn. Churchill Livingstone-Elsevier, Edinburgh.

Leeb, B.F., Schweitzer, H., Montag, K. & Smolen, J. (2000) A meta-analysis of chondroitin sulfate in the treatment of osteoarthritis. *Journal of Rheumatology* **27,** 205–211.

Melzack, R. & Wall, P.D. (1965) Pain mechanisms: a new theory. *Science* **150,** 971.

Millis, D.L., Levine, D. & Taylor, R.A. (2004) *Canine rehabilitation and physical therapy*. Saunders, St Louis, MO.

Millis, D.L. & Levine D. (2014) *Canine rehabilitation and physical therapy*, 2nd edn. Elsevier, Philadelphia, PA.

Shelton, G.D. (2002) Myasthenia gravis and disorders of neuromuscular transmission. *Veterinary Clinics of North America: Small Animal Practice* **32,** 189–206.

Slatter, D. (2003) Intervertebral disc disease. In: Slatter, D. (ed.), *Textbook of small animal surgery*, 3rd edn. W.B. Saunders, Philadelphia; Chapter 81.

Summer-Smith, G. (1993) Gait analysis and orthopaedic examination. In: Slatter, D. (ed.), *Textbook of small animal surgery*, 2nd edn. W.B. Saunders, Philadelphia; p. 1578.

Tator, C.H. & Fehlings, M.G. (1991) Review of the secondary injury theory of acute spinal cord trauma with emphasis on vascular mechanisms. *Journal of Neurosurgery* **75,** 15–26.

Yarrow, T.G. & Jeffery, N.D. (2000) Dura mater laceration associated with acute paraplegia in three dogs. *Veterinary Record* **146,** 138–139.

Self-assessment answers

Chapter 1: Musculoskeletal physiotherapy

1 In cases of hip dysplasia, which passive movement of the coxofemoral (hip) joint is usually most restricted and painful?
b Extension

2 If an animal is 5/5 lame in the left pelvic limb for more than 2 weeks, what changes can be expected in the affected limb?
a Generalised muscle atrophy, tight hip flexors, and weak hamstrings.

3 Incomplete ossification of the humeral condyle (IOHC) is a condition mostly seen in:
d Springer spaniels

4 When considering the pain gate control theory, which of the following would lead to pain perception in the brain?
c C fibre stimulation

5 Which of the following inhibits pain perception in the brain?
b A-beta fibres

6 Which of the following is not considered to be a strengthening exercise?
d Passive range of motion exercises

Practical Physiotherapy for Veterinary Nurses, First Edition. Donna Carver.

7 When using which piece of electrotherapy, must dark-green lens glasses be worn for eye protection?
b Laser machine

8 Which of the following is not a naturally occurring opioid?
a Methadone

9 Which exercise would most challenge a patient's balance?
d Patient standing with all four limbs on a moving wobble board.

10 What is the sequence of cranial cruciate disease events?
a Stifle instability, articular cartilage degeneration, capsular fibrosis, reduced ROM.

Chapter 2: Neurology

1 PROM exercises are predominantly performed to:
b Maintain joint ROM in the affected limbs

2 Stretching muscles aims to:
a Maintain or improve muscle length

3 In which of the following situations might hydrotherapy be contraindicated?
c The patient currently has a urinary tract infection

4 Tetraparesis is a term used to describe:
d Weakness in all four limbs.

5 Where would you localise a lesion to in a tetraparetic patient?
a C1-C5

6 Which cranial nerves control pupil size and can be stimulated by light?
a 2, 3

7 Myasthenia gravis is classified as a:
a Neuromuscular disease

8 How would a fibrocartilaginous embolism (FCE) be classified?
d Vascular

9 Which exercise would best challenge/improve proprioception?
b Cavaletti poles

10 Which position should a patient be in when assessing muscle tone?
c A side lying position.

Chapter 3: Respiratory physiotherapy

1 When would manual techniques (percussion, vibrations, etc.) be contraindicated?
c Pneumothorax

2 Which of the following ABG results would indicate an uncompensated respiratory acidosis?
a pH decreased; P_aCO_2 increased; HCO_3 normal.

3 Which of the following ABG results would indicate a compensated respiratory acidosis?
a pH normal; P_aCO_2 increased; HCO_3 increased.

4 What is a normal inspiratory/expiratory respiratory ratio?
d 1:2

5 In a patient with COPD how would the inspiratory/expiratory ratio change?
d 1:3

6 When auscultating a chest which condition would you associate with fine end-of-inspiration crackles?
d Pulmonary oedema

7 Which of the following conditions would benefit from manual physiotherapy techniques (percussion and vibrations)?
c Bronchitis

8 Which of the following conditions is not classified as COPD?
 c Pneumonia

9 Which of the following equations measures cardiac output (CO)?
 c CO = HR × SV

10 Which of the following is used to measure hypoxia?
 b P_aO_2

Chapter 4: Hydrotherapy

1 What is the optimum hydrotherapy pool pH level range?
 d 7.2–7.6

2 What is the optimum hydrotherapy pool bromine level range?
 c 2–6 ppm

3 What is the optimum hydrotherapy pool temperature?
 a 30°C

4 When using a UWT which variable should be adjusted to increase stride length?
 c Increase treadmill belt speed.

5 Which variable will increase the patient's buoyancy when using a UWT?
 d Increasing the water level.

6 When using a UWT at what level is there most resistance from the water?
 a At the surface level of the water.

7 When treating a patient with hip dysplasia, at what level should the water be set to optimise patient strength?
 c At the level of the proximal femur.

8 When treating a patient with elbow dysplasia, at what level should the water be set to optimise patient strength?
b At a level just above the elbow joint.

9 Which one of the following would be considered a caution when carrying out hydrotherapy in a UWT?
a The patient gas a grade II heart murmur; he is not currently on any medication for this.

10 Which one of the following would not be considered a contraindication when carrying out hydrotherapy in a UWT?
d The patient has had sutures removed from a healed surgical incision site the day before.

Index

Practical Physiotherapy for Veterinary Nurses, First Edition. Donna Carver.

Printed and bound by CPI Group (UK) Ltd, Croydon, CR0 4YY

27/10/2024

14580210-0001